BACK TO PROTEIN

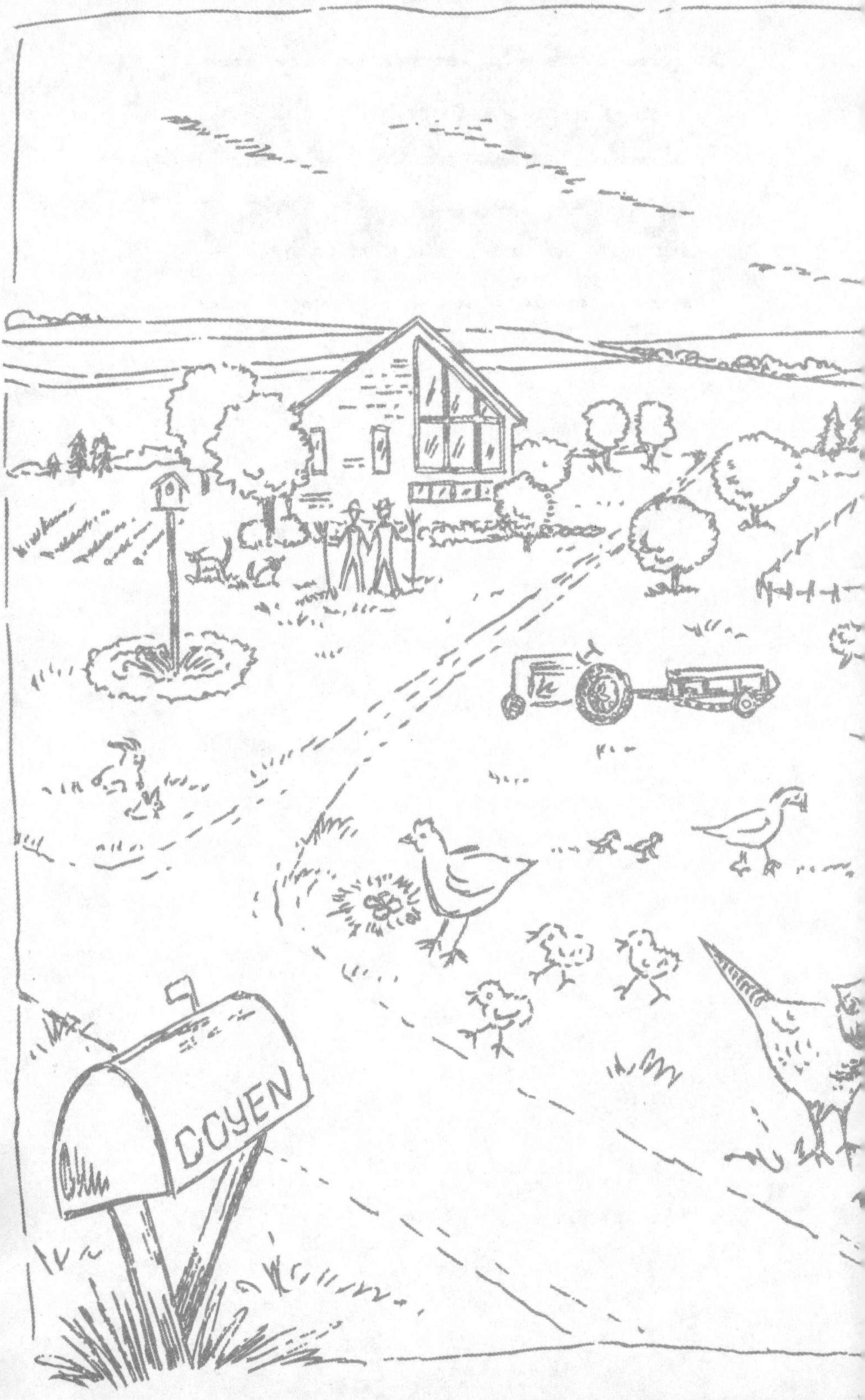
DOYEN

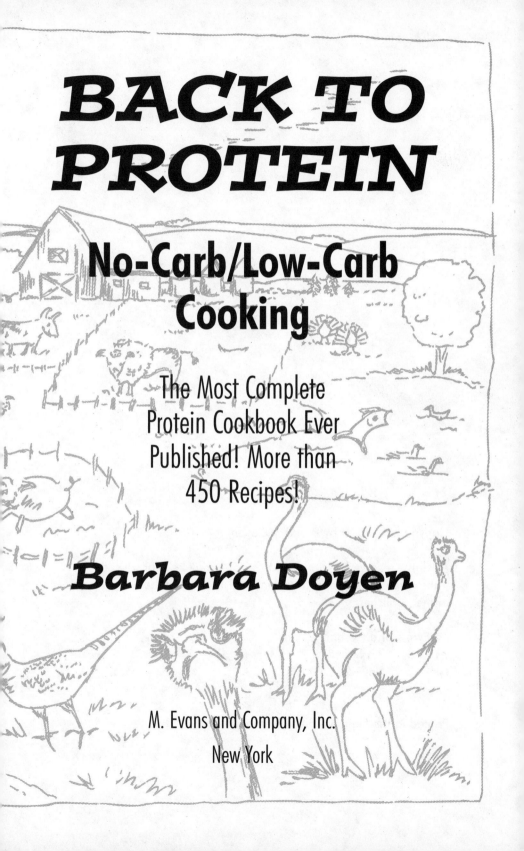

BACK TO PROTEIN

No-Carb/Low-Carb Cooking

The Most Complete
Protein Cookbook Ever
Published! More than
450 Recipes!

Barbara Doyen

M. Evans and Company, Inc.

New York

M. Evans and Company, Inc.
216 East 49th Street
New York, New York 10017

Printed in the United States of America

9 8 7 6 5 4 3 2 1

If you are tired of seeing hundreds of vegetarian cookbooks published year after year and long for something different,
this book is for you!

If you are interested in new ways to cook protein but don't know where to begin,
this book is for you!

If you are on a protein-based diet but are bored with the same plain meat dishes and yearn for new taste sensations,
this book is for you!

With more than 450 recipes and countless variations for the recipes, you'll find a wealth of new taste treats and never be bored again!

On a protein-based diet but hate giving up the foods you love?
Back to Protein shows you how to have all the great taste without the carbs.

You can make fantastic
- *Lasagna*—without pasta
- *Pizzas*—without the crust
- *Chicken Enchilada*—without the shells
- *Quiche*—without the crust
- *Beef Stroganoff*—without noodles
- *Crusted Beef Wellington*—without pastry
- *Sloppy Joes*—without a sugar sauce
- *Taco salad meat*—without a packaged mix
- *"BLT" Chicken*—without the bread
- *Chimichangas*—without tortillas
- *Crunchy Chicken Breast Strips*—without the breading

High-Energy, Low- or No-Carbohydrate Recipes with
- No sugar
- No refined flour
- No artificial sweeteners (except for two recipes)

THE MOST COMPLETE PROTEIN COOKBOOK EVER WRITTEN!
Over 40 recipes for burgers! Over 27 ground beef dishes! 13 beef stews! 14 beef roasts! 48 steak recipes! 59 pork! 95 chicken! 29 turkey! 53 fish and seafood! 20 lamb! 22 Exotic recipes using alligator, bison, etc., plus many others, including numerous variations.

I have a friend who absolutely never would serve a new recipe to guests without testing it first.

I am not like that.

My husband calls me his "creative cook." Even when I have a recipe perfected, I cannot resist tweaking it, experimenting with this or that new combination or technique to make it better or different.

My husband has often requested a dish he particularly enjoyed, only to have me tell him I can't remember how I made it, to his disappointment. For years, his favorite comment at meal time became "This is great—did you write it down?" And when I repeatedly answered "no," he'd turn to the kids and say "We'd better enjoy this, because we're never having it again!"

Well, I finally started to write it down. This book is the result.

And so I'd like to dedicate it, with great love, and much laughter, to my wonderful husband, Bob Doyen.

Contents

Chapter 8
EXOTIC MEATS: Alligator, Bison, Deer, Duck, Goose, Ostrich,

Introduction

"It's amazing that you and Bob haven't gained a lot of weight," say friends who've heard I'm writing a cookbook and sometimes preparing three or four protein dishes at a meal.

Actually, nothing could be further from the truth. Quite the opposite.

You can eat all the food in this cookbook, in quantities that will satisfy you, without running the risk of getting fat. But that wasn't the reason for this book.

I developed these recipes for health. Bob's and mine. And yours, dear reader, if you have the courage to sort through all the food misinformation out there.

So how did a near-vegetarian who doesn't even particularly like meat end up on a solidly protein diet?

As the head of my own literary agency, I've sold excellent vegetarian books. I adore vegetables and fruits, grains and legumes in all their forms. For eight years I cooked near vegetarian meals with low amounts of animal protein and extremely low amounts of fat because Bob's doctors told us we had to do this to combat his high blood pressure and cholesterol. In addition, I've had a lifelong problem with low blood sugar; doctors told me the answer was to eat a high carb diet with frequent snacks. Always underweight, I was even advised to eat a large malt daily to gain weight! (I love malts and was glad to try, but I didn't gain weight and instead felt quite sick from all the sugar.) And then, as I approached middle age and became really strict about fat restriction for Bob's health, weight began to appear—a little too much weight. Worse, I never had energy and felt so ill all the time I was afraid I'd become an invalid.

It was time to take charge of my own health.

A book person, and a thorough researcher, I knew the answer had to be out there, and in print, if I only knew where to look. For the first time, I began to read all those weight- loss books that never seemed appropriate for me before. Not to lose weight but to find health.

I read many books and medical journal articles. Finally, I came to *Dr. Atkins' New Diet Revolution*, which has literally changed my life!

• I learned that there are three macro nutrients: fat, protein, and carbohydrates. (All the vitamins and minerals are considered micronutrients.) If you restrict fat and protein, all you have left to live on are the carbohydrates. And the carbs cause an insulin response that results in all kinds of health problems, particularly when the carbs come from refined flours and sugars.

• I learned that there are numerous studies documenting the body's requirement of essential fatty acids and essential amino acids, which come from fat and protein, but there is no such thing as an essential carbohydrate!

• I learned that eating fat doesn't make you fat; eating carbohydrates does!

• I learned that eating fat and meat and eggs doesn't give you heart trouble or high cholesterol or clog your arteries; eating refined flours and sugars does!

So Bob and I are back to eating marbled steak, real butter, and real cream. No more fear of fat! Now we eat liberal amounts of eggs and all kinds of meats—we're *back to protein!* And we both feel great—and so do the many others we've introduced to this way of eating.

There was only one problem—a protein-centered diet is easy to follow, but quickly becomes boring unless one has access to hundreds of fabulous recipes. But I couldn't find a satisfying protein cookbook. So I wrote it myself.

This is the most complete protein cookbook ever published!

Barbara Doyen

Author's Note

To make this book ultra easy to read and to use:

- All ingredients are listed in the order they're used.
- Dry ingredients are listed before wet ingredients to reduce the need for duplicate measuring cups and spoons.
- Ingredients that go together in one step are grouped together.
- Most recipes are formulated to serve one or two people and are easily multiplied.
- Variations for many recipes are included in an "Options" section.
- Each protein is in its own chapter; recipes for each cut are arranged together and then sorted by cooking method.
- Recipes for leftovers or cooked proteins are found in "encore" sections at the end of each chapter.
- Food safety tips precede each protein along with charts about cooking temperatures and storage times for that protein.

Most recipes take minutes of preparation time, many take less than 30 minutes from starting to eating. To save even more time, cook more than needed to be reheated for later meals.

With the more complicated gourmet recipes, I've simplified the steps as much as possible while still retaining the qualities of the dish. The goal is to have great food prepared as easily as possible.

Need help with measurements and equivalents? It's right after this section: Measurements and Equivalents.

Don't know how to use a meat thermometer? Look right before chapter 1: Using Meat Thermometers.

Entertaining and want no-carb/low-carb appetizers? Check out Appetizer Suggestions and Recipes starting on page 289.

What about no-carb/low-carb salad dressings? Eleven recipes plus variations are found in Encore Salad Basics, page 291.

Want to know where to find the utensils mentioned in preparing the recipe? Contact information is in Equipment Sources: Where to Buy It, page 298.

Where to get ingredients that aren't easily available locally? Find catalogue and web site addresses in Food Sources—Where to Order It, page 300.

Need to know specific carb counts for recipe variations? Consult Carb Counts for the Ingredients, page 302.

FOOD NOTES:

My recipes do not call for the usual prepared prepackaged foods—there is not one can of mushroom soup, not one packet of dried soup mix; nor will you find so-called "lite" margarines or artificial whipped creams—it's far healthier to go for the real thing!

Beware of hidden carbs—convenience foods often include some form of flour or other starch as a thickener and sugar as a flavor enhancement. By cooking your foods from scratch, you also eliminate the over 3,000 different chemical additives and preservatives now present in prepared foods.

Because of the many variables, like how long the meat was marinaded and how absorbent the protein was, or how long the vegetables were cooked, it's very difficult to precisely calculate the carbohydrates in a serving. With the help of a licensed dietician (thanks, Linda!), I've listed the carb count as a range using the following in each recipe:

> **No carbs** = 0 grams carb per serving
> **Trace** = less than 1 gram per serving
> **Very Low carbs** = 5 grams or less per serving
> **Low carbs** = 10 grams or less per serving

The carb counts are for the main recipe; for calculating how a variation alters the carb count, consult the Appendix: Carb Counts for the Ingredients.

Sometimes, cookbook authors use terminology that can be confusing. Please know that:

- A *stalk* of celery is the whole bunch; a *rib* is one stem off the stalk.
- Dry mustard is what you buy in the spice section; prepared mustard is what you use on burgers.
- Ginger is the dry version in cans and jars in the spice section; gingerroot is the fresh tuber that must be peeled before use.
- Herbs and spices in the recipes are the dry form unless specified as fresh.

OTHER MISCELLANEOUS NOTES:

Fresh vs. dried: Fresh herbs and spices are wonderful, but not always available or convenient. If the recipe calls for dried and you want to use fresh, multiply the amount by two or three. When converting the amount of fresh herb or spice to dried, divide by half or one-third.

Countering tomato acid: Never sweeten tomatoes with sugar, not even a pinch; instead add a little carrot, or buy low acid tomatoes. Besides, sugar ruins the taste of tomatoes, in my opinion.

Marinade containers: Use a non reactive pan for marinades with lemon or vinegar or other acid ingredients—use glass or plastic or steel or enamel, not aluminum, which could turn black.

Bouillon cubes have more carbs than bouillon granules, probably because of the binder used to create the cube shape; which is why I recommend using only the granules in my recipes.

Freezing dairy products: You can buy butter on sale and freeze it till needed. Cream cheese can be frozen, too; the texture is somewhat affected but it's still fine for the recipes in this book. You'll never have to worry about mold on your shredded cheese if you store it in the freezer. It's also cheaper in bulk lots of five or ten pounds. Freeze, removing enough shredded cheese to last you about a week; this should be stored in a sealed container in the refrigerator. Blocks of cheese do not freeze well. Never freeze heavy cream.

Westbrae Unsweetened Un-Ketchup is available in health food stores as well as many larger grocery stores across the nation.

Pork Rinds are found in the snack food section of the store, usually with the potato chips.

In addition to a *Cuisinart food processor*, I recommend the *Cuisinart Hand Blender* to blend sauces and dressings as well as to whip heavy cream. It does small jobs well, and—best of all—clean-up is easy!

I love *Cuisinart's PrepBoard cutting surface*. The edges curve up slightly to contain the food and keep liquid from running off, the square size is just right, they're light weight and easy to handle, and the board goes into the dishwasher. I have two—would like four when I'm cooking big meals!

Skillet vs. wok: Although I love my wok, I usually use a large skillet for stir frying simply because my wok won't go into the dishwasher.

Check the labels on everything you buy—you'll be amazed at how many products have added sugar in addition to the natural carbohydrates present in the food. Find alternatives without added sugar.

One last bit of advice: Feel free to write in this cookbook. Note which recipes your family loved, and which variations you tried. *Make this book your indispensable reference guide to cooking fabulous proteins!*

Measurements

I recommend that you buy a set of good measuring spoons and cups. A good set is comfortable to hold, easy to use, and will not flex or warp, distorting the measurement. A great collection contains all the measures listed below. My recipes usually list all the dry ingredients first to prevent the need to wash and dry the measures when switching from liquid to dry ingredients. For convenience, you might want to buy more than one set of measures. The following recipes use these measurements:

- dash = less than ⅛ teaspoon
  Note: Use your own judgment, as there is no "true" measure for a dash. For example, a dash of salt would mean to turn the shaker upside down and quickly right it again; what falls out is a dash.
- pinch = a little more than a dash
  Traditionally, this is the amount you can grasp between your thumb and forefinger; I often use two or three dashes.

- ⅛ teaspoon
- ¼ teaspoon
- ½ teaspoon
- ¾ teaspoon
  or use ¼ teaspoon + ½ teaspoon
- 1 teaspoon
- 1 tablespoon = ½ fluid ounce
- 1½ tablespoons
  or use 1 tablespoon + 1 teaspoon + ½ teaspoon

- ⅛ cup = 2 tablespoons = 1 fluid ounce
- ¼ cup = 4 tablespoons or 2 fluid ounces
- ⅓ cup = 5⅓ tablespoons
  or use 5 tablespoons and 1 teaspoon
- ½ cup = 8 tablespoons
  or use ¼ cup twice

- ⅔ cup = 10⅔ tablespoons
  or use 10 tablespoons + 2 teaspoons or ½ cup + 2 tablespoons + 2 teaspoons
- ¾ cup = 12 tablespoons
  or use ½ cup + ¼ cup
- 1 cup = 16 tablespoons
  or 8 fluid ounces (get both dry and liquid 1-cup measures)
- 1 pint = 2 cups
  or use the 1-cup measure twice
- 1 quart = 4 cups
  or use the 2-cup measure twice
- ½ gallon = 2 quarts = 8 cups
  or use the 4-cup measure twice
- 1 gallon = 4 quarts = 16 cups

OTHER HANDY MEASURES

Eggs
- 2 large or 3 medium eggs measure about ½ cup
- 5 medium eggs measure about 1 cup

Butter
- 1 stick = ½ cup = 4 ounces
- 4 sticks = 2 cups = 1 pound

Cheese
- 4 cups, shredded = 1 pound = 16 ounces
- 2 cups cottage cheese = 1 pound = 16 ounces
- 1 cup Philadelphia cream cheese = 8 ounces
- 3-ounce package Philadelphia cream cheese = 6 tablespoons

Milk
- 1 cup heavy whipping cream yields 2 to 2½ cups whipped cream

Chickens
- 1 broiler = about 3 pounds
- 1 roaster = about 6 pounds

Citrus
- 1 lemon = 3 tablespoons juice
- 1 lemon = about 1½ to 2 teaspoons zest
- 1 lime = about ½ to 1 teaspoons zest
- 1 orange = about 1 tablespoon zest

Nuts

- 1 pound shelled nuts = about 3½ to 4 cups nut meats
- ¼ pound nuts = about 1 cup chopped nuts

Herbs and Spices

- 1 teaspoon dried = 1 tablespoon fresh

Using a Meat Thermometer

Have you ever cut into a roast or a turkey while it's in the oven to see if it has finished cooking? It's an inconvenience, especially if you have to do it several times. Using a meat thermometer takes such guesswork out of cooking. A meat thermometer can also help you:

- Prevent food-borne illnesses
- Prevent overcooking
- Hold foods at a safe temperature.

If you don't regularly use a meat thermometer, you should get into the habit of using one. A meat thermometer measures the internal temperature of your cooked meat and poultry—or even casseroles—to ensure that a safe temperature has been reached and that harmful bacteria such as certain strains of *salmonella* and *E. Coli* have been destroyed.

TYPES OF MEAT THERMOMETERS

• **Regular, ovenproof types** go into the food at the beginning of the cooking time and can be read easily.

• **Instant-read and digital types** are not intended to go in the food while it's in the oven, but will give you a quick reading when inserted into the food; they can be read easily.

• **Pop-up types**, commonly found in poultry, may be purchased for other types of meats. Pop-up thermometers are reliable to within one to two degrees Farenheit if accurately placed in the product. The "pop-up" feature indicates that the food has reached the final temperature for safety and doneness, but it is also suggested that the temperature of the food be checked with a conventional thermometer in several places.

• **Microwave-safe types** are specially designed only for use in microwave ovens.

BUYING TIPS

• Make sure the thermometer you buy is designed for meat and poultry. There are other types of thermometers; for example, candy thermometers. Read the package label carefully to make sure you are buying the type designed for use with meats.
• Look for an easy-to-read dial, made with stainless steel and a shatterproof clear lens.
• Meat thermometers that can be calibrated for accuracy and digital thermometers are also available.

USING A MEAT THERMOMETER

What about accuracy? The accuracy of the meat thermometer can be verified and the thermometer calibrated if necessary. Some thermometers have "test" marks on them at 212° F., the boiling point of water at sea level. To test the thermometer, insert at least two inches of the stem into boiling water. It should read 212 degrees F.

Some thermometers, especially the "instant-read" type, have a recalibration or adjustment nut under the dial. Turn the nut if necessary to adjust. (NOTE: Water boils at a lower temperature at higher altitudes; for example, 202°F at 5,000 feet.)

Where do I insert the thermometer?

Insert the thermometer in the thickest part, away from bone, fat, and gristle.
  • For poultry, insert the thermometer into the inner thigh area near the breast, but not touching the bone.
  • For roasts, steaks, chops, or ground meat, and ground poultry, insert the thermometer into the thickest area. It may be inserted sideways in thin items such as patties.
  • For casseroles, insert the thermometer into the thickest portion.

When do I insert the thermometer?

Use the following guidelines:
  • An oven-proof thermometer may be inserted into the food at the beginning of the cooking time and remain there throughout cooking. The temperature indicator will rise as the food cooks.

Back to Protein

• Instant-read thermometers are not designed to stay in the food during cooking. If you are using an instant-read thermometer, pull the meat or poultry out of the oven far enough to insert the stem about two inches into the thickest part of the food but not touching bone. The temperature should register in about fifteen seconds.

CLEAN-UP

After each use, wash the stem section of the meat thermometer thoroughly in hot, soapy water.

—From a brochure by the Iowa State University Extension, with the U.S. Department of Agriculture.

Chapter 1

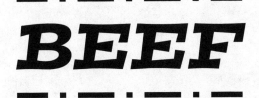

W e live smack dab in the center of the richest farm country in the world where nearly every farmstead once had its own cattle herd numbering from a few dozen to a few hundred head. My husband kept his herd in pasture ground by the Racoon River for many years, riding horseback to sort them for market, to check on his cows during calving season, or to bottle-feed a calf in trouble. I am the animal-lover, but even Bob has a soft spot in his heart for a newborn calf.

Sadly, the farm crisis of the 1980s forced many Midwestern farmers out of the cattle business—some out of farming altogether; plummeting prices caused many others to abandon cattle entirely, my husband included. For years I used his leftover hay bales as mulch on my garden. Last year, when butter went up to about five dollars a pound, I suggested perhaps we should consider getting a milk cow, but Bob just shook his head and gave me one of his "You're crazy, woman!" looks.

We get our beef cuts from local butchers, and it's all high-quality, as you might expect. We especially like the Top of Iowa steaks from our nearby store. Their rump roasts are excellent, as is their lean stew meat, already cut into cubes and ready to use. The ground beef we get from our hometown locker is unsurpassed; I never have to worry about grease in the skillet—thanks, Bruce! When you buy ground beef for the recipes that follow, try to get the leanest possible. And when cooking crumbled ground beef on the stove, if you find you have much grease, pour it out before proceeding with the recipe.

SAFETY TIPS FOR BEEF

• The Iowa State University Extension recommends that all beef should be cooked to 160°F (for medium) or 170° (for well-done). Meat is ready when it is brown or gray inside.

• Be sure to cook ground beef adequately to destroy bacteria. Ground beef should be brown or gray in the center. Meatloaf should cook to an internal temperature of 170°F.

• Don't cross contaminate. When cooking meat on the grill, make sure the plate used to carry the raw meat to the grill is washed thoroughly before using it to bring cooked meat to the table.

• The Iowa State University Extension advises that when reheating leftovers such as chili, lasagna, or casseroles, bake or cook them until a meat thermometer reads 140° or higher, or until the mixture is hot and bubbly throughout.

• Store ground beef in the coldest part of the refrigerator or wrap securely and freeze.

• Thaw beef and ground beef in the refrigerator.

• When thawing in the refrigerator, always place the meat on a plate or a pan to so juices do not contaminate other food. Raw juices often contain bacteria.

BEEF STORAGE TIMES

	Refrigerated at 40°F	Frozen at 0°F or colder
Hamburger and stew meats	1 to 2 days	3 to 4 months
Steak	3 to 5 days	6 to 12 months
Roasts	3 to 5 days	6 to 12 months
Leftover meat and meat dishes	3 to 4 days	2 to 3 months

Back to Protein

INTERNAL COOKED TEMPERATURE FOR BEEF

Ground beef   160°F (Cook until no longer pink.)
Roasts and steaks
    Medium   160°F
    Well-done   170°F

Never serve meat that has been cooked rare (less than 145°F). Refer to "Using Meat Thermometers" on page xviii.

(Information courtesy of Iowa State University Extension)

MAKING BURGERS: AN IMPORTANT NOTE

In order to handle the meat as little as possible, use a rubber spatula to scrape the ground beef mixtures from the sides of the mixing bowl and shape into a ball. Use the spatula as a knife to cut the ball. Shape and flatten the desired number of burgers, handling as little as possible. Place the patties on waxed paper until ready to cook.

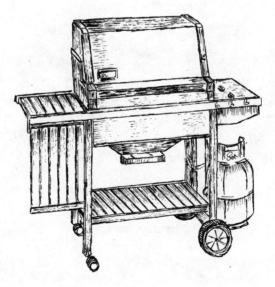

Basic Burgers

1 pound ground beef
1 egg

Salt and pepper (optional)

1. Preheat an outdoor grill on high OR preheat a broiler to high OR melt 1 tablespoon butter in a skillet on the stove on low heat.
2. Combine all of the ingredients in a mixer with a flat paddle beater on the lowest setting for 10 seconds OR mix together by hand until just blended. Do not overmix.
3. Shape into burger patties.
4. Place the burgers on the grill. Turn the heat down to medium OR broil on high heat, watching carefully, OR increase heat to medium and add the burgers to the skillet.
5. Turn the burgers when brown on one side.
6. When both sides are browned and the meat is no longer pink inside, remove from the heat and serve with desired condiments.

OPTIONS
• Pour a little red wine in the skillet while frying the burgers.
• Serve the burgers with Westbrae Unsweetened Un-Ketchup, prepared mustard, a few dill chips, or a little diced onion for a very low-carb burger.

> To keep the carbohydrates low, serve all the burger recipes without hamburger buns.

Walnut Curry Burgers

1 pound hamburger
1 egg
2 to 3 tablespoons walnut pieces
1 to 2 teaspoons curry powder

1 tablespoon butter

1. Combine the hamburger, egg, walnuts, and curry powder in a mixer with a flat beater or dough hook on the lowest setting until ingredients are just mixed. (I use a KitchenAid® mixer on "1" setting). Shape into burger patties.
2. Melt the butter in a medium skillet.

3. Place the burgers in the skillet. Cook until all the meat is gray, with no pink inside.

OPTIONS

• These burgers are fabulous when cooked on the grill. If desired, you can top each burger with a pat of butter before serving.

COMMENTS

This wonderful recipe was inspired by one in Dr. and Mrs. Atkins' cookbook.

• Since I often eat these burgers for breakfast, I usually cook more than one pound of burgers at a time and then refrigerate the extras for reheating in the microwave for future breakfasts.

Barbecue Burgers

VERY LOW CARBOHYDRATES   **NUMBER OF SERVINGS: 2**

> *1 pound ground beef*
> *2 tablespoons Westbrae Unsweetened Un-*
> *   Ketchup*
> *1 tablespoon dried minced onion*
> *1 teaspoon prepared mustard*
> *1 teaspoon prepared horseradish*
> *1 teaspoon Worcestershire Sauce*
> *Dash black pepper*

1. Preheat grill on high.
2. Combine all of the ingredients in a mixer with a flat paddle beater on the lowest setting for 10 seconds OR mix together by hand until just blended. Do not overmix.

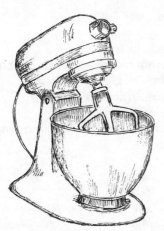

3. Shape into burger patties. Place the burgers on the grill. Reduce heat to medium and cook until all the meat is gray with no pink left inside.

OPTIONS

• Place the burgers on a broiler pan coated with vegetable oil spray and broil to desired doneness, turning meat when half done. OR melt 1 to 2 tablespoons of butter in a skillet and pan fry to desired doneness, turning once.

Walnut Burgers
with Soy Sauce

VERY LOW CARBOHYDRATES   **NUMBER OF SERVINGS: 2**

1 pound ground beef
1 egg
⅓ cup chopped walnuts
2 small chopped green onions, including
*   tops*
1 tablespoon no-carb soy sauce, such as
*   Kikkoman's*
¼ teaspoon black pepper
1 tablespoon butter or olive oil (optional)

1. Combine all of the ingredients in a mixer with a flat paddle beater on the lowest setting for 10 seconds OR mix together by hand until just blended. Do not overmix.
2. Shape into burger patties.
3. Fry in butter on medium heat, OR grill on medium heat OR broil on high heat, watching carefully.

OPTIONS

• Consider varying the shape of the burgers. For instance, since I'm usually cooking for two, I might make the burgers oblong to fit into a small skillet.

Wine Burgers

VERY LOW CARBOHYDRATES   **NUMBER OF SERVINGS: 4 OR 5**

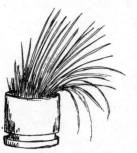

2 pounds ground beef
1 egg
3 tablespoons red cooking wine
2 tablespoons finely chopped fresh or 2 tea-
*   spoons dried chives, sage, parsley,*
*   thyme, or a combination of these*
1 tablespoon Dijon mustard
½ teaspoon black pepper (up to 1 teaspoon,
*   if desired)*
Salt as desired

1. Pre-heat grill on high.
2. Combine all of the ingredients in a mix with a flat paddle beater on the lowest setting for 10 seconds OR mix by hand. Do not overmix.

3. Shape into burger patties.
4. Place burgers on the grill and turn the heat down to medium OR broil or fry in a skillet with 2 tablespoons of butter. Cook until all the meat is gray with no pink left inside.

> I grow chives in a flowerpot on my kitchen windowsill year round, so when a recipe calls for fresh chives, I just snip off what I need.

Barbecue Beer Burgers

VERY LOW CARBOHYDRATES   **NUMBER OF SERVINGS: 4 OR 5**

2 pounds ground beef
1 egg
¼ cup Miller Lite Beer (Additional ¼ cup for basting)
3 tablespoons dried minced onion
1 clove garlic, minced
1 teaspoon Tabasco Sauce (I use the mild)
1 teaspoon chili powder
1 teaspoon beef bouillon granules
⅛ teaspoon black pepper

1. Preheat grill or broiler on high.
2. Combine the ingredients in a mixer with a flat paddle beater on the lowest setting for 10 seconds OR mix by hand. Do not overmix.
3. Shape into burger patties.
4. Grill or broil, basting with the additional beer.

OPTIONS
• You can serve these burgers with low-carb salsa.

Dilly Burgers

VERY LOW CARBOHYDRATES   **NUMBER OF SERVINGS: 2**

1 tablespoon butter
1 pound ground beef

½ cup sour cream
1½ teaspoons dill seed OR 1½ tablespoons
*   fresh dill weed*
½ teaspoon prepared mustard
Salt and pepper as desired

1. Shape into burger patties and fry with the butter in a skillet OR grill OR broil them.
2. Combine the sour cream, mustard, dill, salt and pepper and spoon on top of the burgers.

OPTIONS

- Melt the butter in a skillet. Add the beef and cook on medium heat till browned, then add the sour cream, mustard, dill, salt and pepper. Heat through and serve.

Philly Burgers

VERY LOW CARBOHYDRATES   **NUMBER OF SERVINGS: 2**

1 pound ground beef
¼ cup Philadelphia Cream Cheese (not
*   "lite" or "reduced fat"); bring to room*
*   temperature*
2 tablespoons diced chives OR a finely
*   diced onion OR a combination of the*
*   two.*
Pepper as desired
Extra cream cheese for topping, if desired

1. Preheat grill on high.
2. Combine all of the ingredients in a mixer with a flat paddle beater on the lowest setting for 10 seconds OR mix by hand. Do not overmix.
3. Shape into burger patties.
4. Grill OR fry in a skillet with 1 tablespoon butter or olive oil.
5. Serve with an additional dollop of cream cheese, if desired.

OPTIONS

Instead of using cream cheese, try using sour cream, combined with a French onion dip—but be sure to check the carbs.

         Back to Protein

Pimento-Mushroom Burgers

VERY LOW CARBOHYDRATES **NUMBER OF SERVINGS: 2**

1 tablespoon butter
1 cup diced mushrooms
2 tablespoons finely chopped onion
1 tablespoon finely minced celery
1 tablespoon chopped pimento

1 pound ground beef
1 egg
2 tablespoons minced fresh parsley
2 teaspoons Worcestershire sauce
¼ teaspoon salt
Dash black pepper

1 or 2 tablespoons low-carb salsa, if desired, for topping

1. Preheat grill or broiler on high.
2. Melt the butter in a small skillet and add the mushrooms, onion, celery, and pimento. Cook on low heat, allowing the liquid to evaporate.
3. Combine the mushroom mixture with the beef, egg, parsley, Worcestershire sauce, salt, and pepper in a mixer with a flat paddle beater on the lowest setting for 10 seconds OR mix by hand. Do not overmix.
4. Shape into burgers patties.
5. Coat the grill rack with vegetable oil spray and turn the heat down to medium. Serve with salsa if desired.

Lemon-Spice Burgers

VERY LOW CARBOHYDRATES   **NUMBER OF SERVINGS: 2**

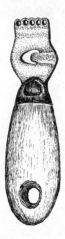

1 pound ground beef
1 teaspoon lemon zest
1 teaspoon lemon juice
½ teaspoon instant beef bouillon granules
½ teaspoon sage
½ teaspoon dry ginger
⅛ teaspoon black pepper
1 or 2 drops Tabasco (we prefer the mild)

1. Combine all of the ingredients in a mixer with a flat paddle beater on the lowest setting for 10 seconds OR mix by hand. Do not overmix.
2. Shape into burger patties.
3. Broil OR grill OR pan fry in 1 or 2 tablespoons of butter or olive oil.

Always wash the skins of your lemons, limes, and even oranges before removing the zest (the outer colored layer, not the white pith beneath) and squeezing for the juice. Zest can be placed in small plastic bags and frozen for later use. Zest adds a nice flavoring to many proteins.

Horseradish Burgers

VERY LOW CARBOHYDRATES   **NUMBER OF SERVINGS: 2**

1 pound ground beef
2 tablespoons Westbrae Unsweetened Un-Ketchup
1 tablespoon minced dried onion
1½ teaspoons prepared mustard
1 teaspoon horseradish
1 teaspoon Worcestershire Sauce
Salt and pepper as desired

1. Combine all ingredients in a mixer with flat paddle beater on lowest setting for 10 seconds OR mix by hand. Do not over handle the meat.
2. Shape into burger patties.
3. Broil OR grill OR pan fry in 1 or 2 tablespoons of butter or olive oil.

Bob's Favorite
Chili Burgers

NUMBER OF SERVINGS: 2

1 pound ground beef
1 egg
¼ cup diced black olives
1 teaspoon chili powder (or more to taste)

Salt and pepper to taste

1. Combine all of the ingredients in a mixer with a flat paddle beater on the lowest setting for 10 seconds OR mix by hand. Do not overmix.
2. Shape into burger patties.
3. Broil OR grill OR pan fry in 1 or 2 tablespoons of butter or olive oil.

OPTIONS
• Serve topped with a dollop of sour cream and/or shredded cheddar cheese.

Barb's Favorite
Chili Burgers

LOW CARBOHYDRATES NUMBER OF SERVINGS: 2

1 pound ground beef
1 egg
¼ cup diced black olives
1 teaspoon lemon zest
1 clove garlic, minced
½ teaspoon chili powder (or more to taste)
½ teaspoon Dijon mustard
¼ teaspoon basil
¼ teaspoon oregano

Salt and pepper as desired

1. Combine all of the ingredients in a mixer with a flat paddle beater on the lowest setting for 10 seconds OR mix by hand. Do not overmix.
2. Turn meat out on waxed paper, divide and shape into patties.
3. Broil OR grill OR pan fry in 1 or 2 tablespoons of butter or olive oil.

OPTIONS
• Serve topped with a dollop of sour cream and/or shredded cheddar cheese.

Burgers with Mushroom Topping

2 pounds ground beef
1 egg
⅓ cup finely chopped onion
1 teaspoon lemon zest OR ½ teaspoon gran-
*   ulated lemon peel*
1 teaspoon beef bouillon granules
1 teaspoon Kitchen Bouquet (3 grams carb)
*   OR Worcestershire sauce (no grams carb)*
1 teaspoon dried parsley flakes
½ teaspoon black pepper

3 tablespoons butter
½ pound mushrooms, sliced
2 teaspoons Dijon mustard

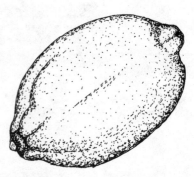

1. Combine beef, egg, onion, zest or peel, bouillon, Kitchen Bouquet or sauce, parsley, and black pepper in a mixer with a flat paddle beater on the lowest setting for 10 seconds OR mix by hand. Do not overmix.
2. Shape into burger patties.
3. While broiling OR grilling OR pan frying in 1 or 2 tablespoons of butter or olive oil, make the mushroom topping. Melt the butter in a skillet. Add the mushrooms and stir fry on medium heat until cooked and the moisture has evaporated. Add the Dijon and stir together.
4. Serve the burgers with the mushroom topping.

Italian Stuffed Burgers

1 pound ground beef OR ½ pound ground
*   beef plus ½ pound bulk pork sausage*
1 egg
Dash pepper (optional)

Several slices pepperoni, chopped
4 or 5 black olives, chopped
3 or 4 tablespoons shredded mozzarella cheese
½ to 1 teaspoon of Italian herb blend
1 tablespoon grated Parmesan cheese
(optional)

1. Preheat grill on high OR preheat broiler to high OR melt 1 tablespoon butter in an ovenproof skillet on the stove on low while preparing the meat.
2. Combine meat, egg, and pepper in mixer with a flat paddle beater on the lowest setting for 10 seconds OR mix together by hand until just blended. Do not overmix.
3. Shape into burger patties on individual squares of waxed paper.
4. Divide the pepperoni, olives, mozzarella, and herbs between the two burgers. Place the stuffing only on one half of each patty, to within 1/4 inch of the outer edges. Using the waxed paper as an aid, gently fold the burger in half. Carefully seal the edges so the stuffing won't leak out. The burgers will be in the shape of a half circle.
5. Melt 2 tablespoons butter in a small, ovenproof skillet. Peel back the waxed paper from one side and carefully place the burger in the butter, with the curved edge to the outside of the pan. Repeat for the other burger. Cook on medium.
6. When the bottom half of the burgers are done, remove the skillet from the stove and place under the broiler to brown the top. Watch carefully so the burgers don't burn.
7. Serve when both sides are browned and meat is no longer pink inside.

OPTIONS

Top each burger with 1 tablespoon Westbrae Unsweetened Un-Ketchup and sprinkle additional mozzarella and/or Parmesan cheeses on top. Broil for another few seconds until cheese is melted and slightly browned.

Although the directions look lengthy, this recipe can be ready to serve in less than 30 minutes!

Apple Curry Burgers

                    NUMBER OF SERVINGS: 2

1 pound ground beef
1 egg
½ small apple, peeled and diced
¼ cup diced onion
½ teaspoon curry powder
¼ teaspoon garlic powder
¼ teaspoon salt (optional)
¼ teaspoon pepper (optional)
1 ½ teaspoons horseradish
1 teaspoon Dijon mustard
1 to 2 tablespoons butter

1. Combine all of the ingredients except the butter in a mixer with a flat paddle beater on the lowest setting for 10 seconds OR mix together by hand until just blended. Do not overmix.
2. Shape into patties and pan fry in butter until done OR grill or broil OR shape into a loaf, place in baking pan, and bake in the oven at 350° about 45 minutes, or till done. Serve.

Pizza Burgers

VERY LOW CARBOHYDRATES   **NUMBER OF SERVINGS: 2**

1 egg (optional)
½ pound ground beef
½ pound bulk pork sausage
¼ cup finely chopped onion (optional)

2 or more tablespoons Westbrae
       Unsweetened Un-Ketchup
pizza spice blend
1 tablespoon Parmesan cheese
2 slices mozzarella cheese and 2 slices
provolone cheese
OR shredded mozzarella- provolone blend

1. Preheat outdoor grill on high OR preheat broiler to high OR melt 1 tablespoon butter in a skillet on the stove on low heat while preparing the meat.
2. Combine the egg, beef, pork sausage, and onion in a mixer with a flat paddle beater on the lowest setting for 10 seconds OR mix together by hand until just blended. Do not overmix.

3. Shape into burger patties.
4. Cook the burgers on a covered grill (close the lid and reduce the heat to medium) OR place on broiler pan OR fry in butter in a skillet on the stove.
5. Remove from heat and top each burger with Un-Ketchup, a generous sprinkle of pizza seasoning, the Parmesan cheese, and top with the mozzarella and provolone. Place under the broiler to melt the cheese slightly, then serve.

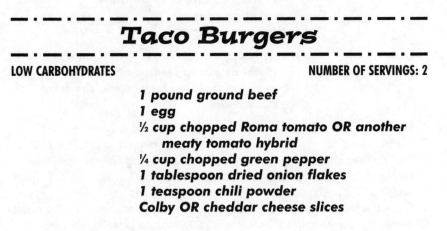

Taco Burgers

LOW CARBOHYDRATES   **NUMBER OF SERVINGS: 2**

1 pound ground beef
1 egg
½ cup chopped Roma tomato OR another
*   meaty tomato hybrid*
¼ cup chopped green pepper
1 tablespoon dried onion flakes
1 teaspoon chili powder
Colby OR cheddar cheese slices

1. Preheat grill on high.
2. Combine all of the ingredients except the cheese in a mixer with a flat paddle beater on the lowest setting for 10 seconds OR mix together by hand until just blended. Do not over mix.
3. Shape into burger patties.
4. Cook the burgers on a covered grill (close the lid and reduce the heat to medium) until all the meat is gray with no pink left inside.
5. Top the hot burgers with cheese and serve.

OPTIONS
• Cook under the broiler OR fry in a skillet with 1 tablespoon butter.

Southwest Burgers

VERY LOW CARBOHYDRATES NUMBER OF SERVINGS: 1

1 pound ground beef
1 egg
1 jalapeno chili pepper, chopped OR ⅓ of a
*   4.5-ounce can chili peppers*
½ teaspoon cumin
Dash black pepper

¼ cup chopped tomato
½ cup thinly sliced lettuce of choice
1 cup shredded Monterey Jack/cheddar
*   cheese blend*

1. Preheat grill on high.
2. Combine beef, egg, chili pepper, cumin and pepper in a mixer with a flat paddle beater on lowest setting for 10 seconds OR mix together by hand until just blended. Do not overmix.
3. Shape into burger patties.
4. Place the burgers on a covered grill (close the lid and reduce the heat to medium). Cook until all the meat is gray with no pink left inside.
5. Top burgers with tomato, lettuce, and cheese and serve.

OPTIONS

• Serve with a little salsa.
• Cook under the broiler OR fry in skillet with 1 tablespoon butter.

Dilly Cheeseburgers

VERY LOW CARBOHYDRATES NUMBER OF SERVINGS: 2

1 pound ground beef
1 egg
¼ cup diced fresh mushrooms
½ teaspoon dill weed
Salt and pepper as desired

¼ cup Hellman's Original mayonnaise
¼ teaspoon additional dill weed
Dash black pepper

2 lettuce leaves
2 slices brick cheese
2 slices cheddar cheese
2 thin tomato slices

1. Preheat grill on high.
2. Combine beef, egg, mushrooms, dill weed, salt, and pepper in a mixer with a flat paddle beater on the lowest setting for 10 seconds OR mix together by hand until just blended. Do not overmix.
3. Shape into patties.
4. Place burgers on a covered grill, (close the lid and reduce the heat to medium). Cook until all meat is gray with no pink left inside.
5. Combine the mayonnaise, dill weed, and pepper.
6. Top each burger with 1 slice of brick cheese, 1 slice of cheddar, and a tomato slice. Place burger on the lettuce leaf, then spread the mayonnaise mix on top.

OPTIONS
- Cook under the broiler OR fry in skillet with 1 tablespoon butter.

Almond Burgers

VERY LOW CARBOHYDRATES   **NUMBER OF SERVINGS: 2**

> *1 pound ground beef*
> *1 egg*
>
> *Salt and pepper, as desired*
> *Garlic powder, as desired*
> *Dried onion flakes, as desired*
> *2 to 4 tablespoons sliced almonds*
> *4 tablespoons cheese, (Monterey Jack,*
> *   Swiss, or mozzarella)*
> *2 tablespoons olive oil*

1. Set the broiler to high.
2. Combine the beef and egg in a mixer with a flat paddle beater on the lowest setting for 10 seconds OR mix by hand. Do not overmix.
3. Divide the mixture in half, then flatten each half into a large patty ½ inch thick, on its own waxed paper.
4. Top each patty with a dash of salt, pepper, and garlic powder, a generous sprinkle of onion flakes, 1 or 2 tablespoons sliced almonds, and 2 tablespoons of cheese.
5. Using the waxed paper, fold the patty in half. Fold back the waxed paper and seal the edges of the meat. The burgers will now be shaped like half circles.
6. Melt the butter in an ovenproof skillet. Pan fry the burgers, without turning, until the bottom side is browned. Place the skillet under the broiler to brown the top for about 5 minutes, or to desired doneness, and serve.

OPTIONS
- Cook the burgers on the stovetop, turning them gently with a wide spatula.

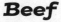

Sesame Burgers

1 pound ground beef
1 egg
· **¼ cup finely chopped onions**
OR 2 tablespoons dried onion flakes
¼ teaspoon salt (or as desired)

¼ cup sesame seeds
2 tablespoons butter

1. Combine the beef, egg, onion, and salt in a mixer with a flat paddle beater on the lowest setting for 10 seconds OR mix by hand. Do not overmix.
2. Shape into burgers. Press 1 tablespoon sesame seeds onto each side of the burgers.
3. Melt the butter in a skillet. Cook the burgers on medium low heat until the meat is no longer pink inside.

OPTIONS
• Substitute celery seed for sesame seed.

This recipe is not suitable for the grill or broiler, as the seeds would burn.

Stuffed Burgers: 12 Variations

1 pound ground beef
1 egg

Stuffing–see variations below

2 tablespoons butter

1. Preheat broiler or convection broiler to high.
2. Combine beef and egg in a mixer with a flat paddle beater on the lowest setting for 10 seconds OR mix together by hand until just blended. Do not overmix.
3. Shape into patties. Place the patties on individual squares of waxed paper.

4. Divide one of the stuffing ingredients between the two burgers. Place the stuffing only on one half of each patty, to within ¼ inch of the outer edges. Use the waxed paper to gently fold the burger in half. Carefully seal the edges of the burger so the stuffing won't leak out. The burger will be in the shape of a half circle.
5. Melt 2 tablespoons butter in a small ovenproof skillet. Peel back the wax paper and carefully place each burger in the butter, with the curved edge to the outside of the pan. Cook on medium.
6. When the bottom half of the burgers are done, remove the skillet from the stove and place under the broiler to brown the top. Watch carefully so the burgers don't burn.
7. When both sides are browned and the meat is no longer pink inside, remove from the broiler and serve.

OPTIONS

Stuffing variations:
- 4 tablespoons sliced green olives stuffed with pimento + 3 tablespoons butter
- 4 tablespoons diced mushrooms (canned or fresh) + 3 tablespoons butter
- 2 tablespoons capers + 2 tablespoons butter
- 4 tablespoons diced mushrooms (canned or fresh) + 4 tablespoons Philadelphia Cream Cheese
- 4 tablespoons sliced green olives stuffed with pimento + 4 tablespoons Philadelphia Cream Cheese
- ¼ cup chopped black olives + 3 tablespoons butter
- 4 tablespoons Philadelphia Cream Cheese + 3 tablespoons diced chives
- 4 tablespoons Philadelphia Cream Cheese + 4 tablespoons chopped green onions, including tops
- 4 tablespoons Philadelphia cream cheese or butter + 2 tablespoons chopped or sliced almonds, walnuts, pecans, or macadamia nuts
- a thick slice or ⅓ cup shredded cheddar, mozzarella, Gouda, or Brie cheese
- 2 large mushrooms and 2 rings green pepper, chopped and cooked together in a little butter + 2 or 3 black olives, chopped
- 2 slices bacon, cooked crisp and crumbled + 2 tablespoons Philadelphia Cream Cheese

> • If you are really good at flipping, you can turn the burgers and brown the other side in the skillet. (I prefer to use the broiler.)
> • This recipe is not a good choice for the outdoor grill, because these burgers tend to fall apart.

Burgers with Cognac and Onion Sauce

LOW CARBOHYDRATES   **NUMBER OF SERVINGS: 2**

1 to 2 tablespoons butter or olive oil
1 pound ground beef

*2 tablespoons finely diced onion OR ½ cup
    chopped green onions,
including tops (about 3 or 4 onions)*
1 tablespoon cognac
2 tablespoons red cooking wine
*2 tablespoons beef broth OR 2 tablespoons
    water plus*
⅛ teaspoon beef bouillon granules

1. Shape the meat into patties. Fry in a skillet with the butter or oil on medium heat, turning once, about 10 minutes total. Meat will be nearly done.
2. If the hamburger is not lean, pour the grease out of the skillet—but do not scrape the skillet. Place the burgers to one side.
3. Add the onions and stir-fry about 30 seconds.
4. Add the cognac, red wine, and beef broth or water and beef bouillon. Cook, reducing liquid somewhat.
5. Serve the burgers topped with onion sauce.

OPTIONS

• As a substitute for the onions—or in addition to the onions—add a 4-ounce can of mushrooms, including the liquid, to the skillet before the cognac, wine, and broth.

This is very quick and easy—and fabulous!

Baked Burgers

LOW CARBOHYDRATES   **NUMBER OF SERVINGS: 2**

1 pound ground beef
1 egg
1 medium onion, chopped
1 medium tomato, chopped
¼ teaspoon black pepper
¼ teaspoon paprika
Salt, as desired

2 tablespoons butter

1. Preheat oven to 400° on bake or 375° for convection bake.
2. Mix all the ingredients together and shape into 2 balls. Place balls in a well-greased baking pan. Make an indentation in the top of each for 1 tablespoon butter. Place butter in wells.
3. Bake or convection bake for 30 minutes or to desired doneness. Serve with favorite condiments.

OPTIONS
• Add ½ of a green pepper, chopped, to the meat mixture before baking.

Broiled Italian Beef Burgers

VERY LOW CARBOHYDRATES   **NUMBER OF SERVINGS: 2 OR MORE**

1 pound ground beef
1½ teaspoons purchased spaghetti spice
*   blend*
½ teaspoon lemon-pepper seasoning
¼ teaspoon onion powder
¼ teaspoon garlic powder
¼ teaspoon black pepper
1 tablespoon lemon juice

2 eggs
1 cup ground pork rinds

1. Preheat broiler or convection broiler to 350°.
2. Combine all of the ingredients except the eggs and pork rinds in a mixer with a flat paddle beater on the lowest setting for 10 seconds OR mix together by hand until just blended. Do not overmix.
3. Divide and shape into patties.
4. Beat eggs with a fork until yolks and whites are blended. Dip burgers into eggs and then roll in the pork rinds.
5. Place on a broiler rack and broil 15 to 20 minutes, or until browned and done.

OPTIONS
• Serve with Westbrae Unsweetened Un-Ketchup.

> **This makes a great appetizer by dividing the meat mixture into 16 small patties and then continuing with steps 4 and 5.**

Hickory Smoked Burgers

NO CARBOHYDRATES 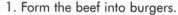 **NUMBER OF SERVINGS: 2**

1 pound ground beef
1 teaspoon Camerons hickory chips

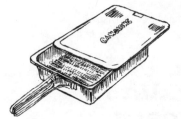

1. Form the beef into burgers.
2. Place the wood chips in the bottom of a Camerons Stovetop Smoker. Place drip tray and rack over the chips. Lay the burgers on the rack.
3. Slide on the lid, leaving it barely cracked open. Place the Smoker on the largest burner on your stove; turn the heat to medium.
4. As soon as you see the first wisp of smoke escape from the Smoker, close the lid and begin timing to 20 minutes. Remove and serve.

OPTIONS

- The smoked burger can be topped with a slice of cheddar cheese and a slice of onion and then smoked for another 2 minutes for a tasty smoked cheeseburger. I sometimes brown the onion in a skillet with a little butter before putting it on the cheese.

One teaspoon of hickory chips will handle up to 3 pounds of ground beef.

Mesquite Smoked Burgers

TRACE OF CARBOHYDRATES **NUMBER OF SERVINGS: 2 TO 4**

½ teaspoon paprika
½ teaspoon cumin
¼ teaspoon garlic powder
¼ teaspoon onion powder
½ teaspoon salt
1 to 2 pounds ground beef, shaped into burgers

1 teaspoon Camerons mesquite wood chips

Pats of butter (optional)
Westbrae Unsweetened Un-Ketchup (optional)

1. Combine the paprika, cumin, garlic powder, onion powder, and salt. Sprinkle over the burgers.

Back to Protein

2. Place the wood chips in the bottom of a Camerons Stovetop Smoker. Place the drip tray and rack over the chips. Lay the burgers on the rack.
3. Slide on the lid, leaving it barely cracked open. Place the Smoker on the largest burner on your stove; turn the heat to medium.
4. As soon as you see the first wisp of smoke escape from the Smoker, close the lid and begin timing to 20 minutes. Do not overcook.
5. If desired, remove the lid and top each burger with a pat of butter. Place the smoker under the broiler a few seconds to melt the butter and lightly brown the burgers. Serve with Westbrae Unsweetened Un-Ketchup.

OPTIONS
• This recipe also works well with Top of Iowa steaks, cut into strips.

Smoked Meatloaf

VERY LOW CARBOHYDRATES   **NUMBER OF SERVINGS: 4**

1 pound ground beef
1 pound ground pork
2 eggs, beaten
½ cup chopped onion
½ cup finely chopped celery
¼ cup chopped parsley
2 cloves garlic, minced
½ teaspoons salt

½ teaspoon Camerons apple wood chips
½ teaspoon Camerons pecan wood chips

1. Combine the meats, eggs, onion, celery, parsley, garlic, and salt. Shape into 2 loaves.
2. Place the wood chips in the bottom of a Camerons Stovetop Smoker. Place the drip tray and rack over the chips. Lay the 2 meat loaves on the rack.
3. Slide on the lid, leaving it barely cracked open. Place the Smoker on the largest burner on your stove; turn the heat to medium.
4. As soon as you see the first wisp of smoke escape from the Smoker, close the lid and begin timing to about 50 minutes.
5. If desired, remove the lid and brush each loaf with 1 tablespoon melted butter. Place the smoker under the broiler for a few seconds until the meat loaves are lightly browned. Remove and serve.

OPTIONS
• Divide the meat into fourths and shape into burgers.

Ground Beef and Hot Dogs

TRACE OF CARBOHYDRATES   **NUMBER OF SERVINGS: 3 OR 4**

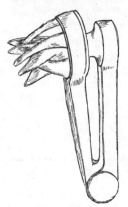

2 tablespoons olive oil
1½ pounds ground beef
4 high quality hot dogs (8 ounces), sliced
   crosswise (check the label for no carbs
   or low carbs and avoid brands with
   added sugar)
1 or 2 cloves of garlic, minced

1. Put the olive oil in a skillet. Cook and crumble the hamburger on medium high heat.
2. Add the sliced hot dogs and minced garlic. Stir fry the mixture until done.

OPTIONS
- Add ⅓ cup chopped onion when frying the hamburger.
- Add 1 teaspoon chili powder to the meat mixture.

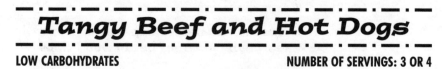

Try topping individual servings with prepared mustard, Westbrae Unsweetened Un-Ketchup, or a little low-carb salsa.

Tangy Beef and Hot Dogs

LOW CARBOHYDRATES   **NUMBER OF SERVINGS: 3 OR 4**

2 tablespoons butter
1 pound ground beef

4 to 8 hot dogs, sliced crosswise
⅓ cup diced green pepper

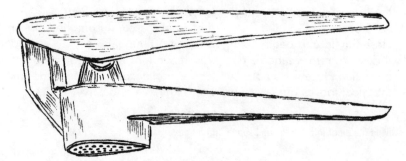

⅓ cup diced onion
⅓ cup diced celery
1 clove garlic, minced

8 ounce can tomato sauce
⅓ cup water or beef bouillon
1 teaspoon dry mustard
½ teaspoon thyme

1. Melt the butter in a skillet. Add beef; stir and crumble till no longer pink.
2. Add the hot dogs, green pepper, onion, celery, and garlic. Cook together till beef is browned and the vegetables are tender.
3. Stir in the tomato sauce, water, or beef bouillion, dry mustard and thyme. Simmer 3 to 5 minutes and serve.

Walnut Curry Hamburger, Loose Meat Style

VERY LOW CARBOHYDRATES   **NUMBER OF SERVINGS: 2**

1 tablespoon butter
2 to 3 tablespoons walnut pieces
1 pound ground beef
1 to 2 teaspoons curry powder

1. Melt the butter in a medium skillet.
2. Add the walnut pieces and stir-fry on medium-low heat for 2 or 3 minutes. Remove the nuts.
3. Add the hamburger to the skillet; stir and crumble until cooked.
4. Sprinkle the meat with the curry powder; stir well.
5. Add the walnuts and serve.

OPTIONS
• Top with a little sour cream.

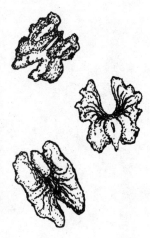

• **This wonderful recipe was inspired by one in Dr. and Mrs. Atkins' cookbook.**
• **I often use this recipe for my breakfast, since it is so quick and easy. I usually prepare more than one pound of hamburger at a time and then refrigerate leftovers for reheating in the microwave for future breakfasts.**

Ground Beef "Teriyaki"

LOW CARBOHYDRATES   **NUMBER OF SERVINGS: 4**

1 or 2 tablespoons oil or butter
2 pounds ground beef
1 cup chopped onion
1 cup green and red pepper strips (half of
    each or all of one)
4 ounces sliced mushrooms (optional)
Gingerroot, about 1 inch diameter and ¼
    inch deep, finely diced OR ¾ teaspoon
    dry ginger
1 garlic clove, minced

2 to 3 tablespoons no carb soy sauce
2 to 3 tablespoons cooking sherry

1. Brown and crumble the hamburger in the oil or butter in a large skillet
   on medium high heat.
2. Add the onion, pepper strips, mushrooms, gingerroot, garlic and stir-
   fry together until the vegetables are done.
3. With the skillet on medium high heat, add the soy sauce and sherry,
   stirring constantly for about one minute. Remove from the stove and
   serve.

This quick and easy recipe takes about 20 minutes total!

Speedy Swedish Meat Balls

LOW CARBOHYDRATES   **NUMBER
                                                OF SERVINGS: 4**

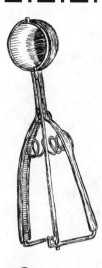

2 pounds ground beef
2 eggs
¼ cup finely chopped onion
½ to 1 teaspoon salt
½ teaspoon nutmeg

¼ cup olive oil

8 ounces Philadelphia Cream Cheese
1 cup cream
¼ cup freshly minced parsley
¼ teaspoon thyme

Back to Protein

1. Combine the beef, eggs, onion, salt, and nutmeg in a mixer, with a flat paddle beater on the lowest setting for 10 seconds. Do not over-mix.
2. Heat the olive oil in a large skillet. Using a 1-inch or a 1 ¼-inch scoop, shape the meatballs and then drop into the skillet. Brown on all sides. Remove the meatballs to a serving bowl; keep warm.
3. Pour off all the liquid from the skillet, but do not scrape the pan. Add the cream cheese, cream, parsley, and thyme. Cook over medium, stirring constantly until the cream cheese is melted and the ingredients are well-mixed. Allow to simmer for a minute or two until thickened.
4. Pour the sauce over the meat balls, coating well: serve.

> It's best to reheat the leftovers in a microwave. If you use the stovetop, reheat meatballs uncovered on low. Do not allow sauce to boil.

Savory Swedish Meat Balls

LOW CARBOHYDRATES   **NUMBER OF SERVINGS: 4 OR MORE**

1 medium onion, finely diced
2 tablespoons butter

1½ pounds lean ground beef
¼ cup heavy cream
1 egg
1 teaspoon salt
1 teaspoon nutmeg
½ teaspoon paprika
½ teaspoon dry mustard
¼ teaspoon pepper

4 tablespoons butter

1 large clove garlic, minced
5 tablespoons butter
½ cup canned double strength beef broth
2 teaspoons Westbrae Unsweetened Un-Ketchup

1 cup sour cream

1. Melt the 2 tablespoons of butter in a skillet; add the onion and cook until transparent.
2. Place the cooked onion, beef, cream, egg, salt, nutmeg, paprika, mustard, and pepper in the bowl of a mixer. Using the flat paddle beater, run the mixer on the lowest speed for 10 seconds to combine the ingredients just until blended. Do not overmix.

3. Melt the 4 tablespoons of butter in a large skillet. Use a 1-inch or 1 ¼-inch scoop to shape the meat into about 48 meatballs. Place in the butter. Brown on all sides. Remove to an ovenproof casserole.
4. Place the minced garlic in the skillet and cook for a few seconds.
5. Add the broth and the Un-Ketchup. Stir on medium heat until thickened. Remove from heat.
6. Place the sour cream in a bowl and gradually add the broth mixture, stirring well.
7. Pour over the meatballs. Stir and serve immediately, or keep warm, uncovered, in a low oven until time to serve.

OPTIONS
• Served as an appetizer or the main course.

• **This recipe takes a bit longer than the previous one, but it's a favorite. It tastes even better the next day—the flavor permeates—so it's a great make-ahead food for entertaining!**
• **When reheating dishes with a cream sauce, like these meatballs, on the stove top, never use a lid—the cream will separate.**

Oriental Meat Balls

LOW CARBOHYDRATES   **NUMBER OF SERVINGS: 2**

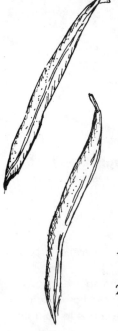

½ *pound ground beef*
½ *pound bulk pork sausage*
1 *tablespoon no carb soy sauce*
1½ *teaspoons vinegar*
1 *clove garlic, minced*
¼ *inch slice gingerroot 1 inch in diameter, finely minced*

2 *tablespoons peanut oil OR olive oil*

1 *cup bean sprouts*
⅓ *cup green pepper strips OR ⅓ cup fresh green beans cut into 1 inch pieces*
4 *ounces sliced mushrooms*

⅓ *cup beef broth*

1. Combine the beef, sausage, soy sauce, vinegar, garlic, and gingerroot.
2. Heat the oil in a wok or a large skillet. Shape 1-inch balls with a dipper and place in hot oil, turning to brown on all sides.
3. Push the meatballs to the side and pour off excess

fat.

4. Add the bean sprouts, green pepper, or green beans and mushrooms and stir fry briefly. Mix the meatballs in with the vegetables.
5. Add the beef broth and simmer 2 minutes until the liquid is reduced a bit. Serve with additional soy sauce, if desired.

The beef broth in my recipes can be homemade, canned, or made from bouillon granules. If I don't have homemade available, either fresh or frozen, I prefer the canned broth.

Parmesan Meatballs

VERY LOW CARBOHYDRATES   **NUMBER OF SERVINGS: 4 AS MAIN COURSE, 20 AS APPETIZER**

1½ pounds ground beef
¾ cup grated Parmesan cheese
2 eggs
1 teaspoon dried parsley
Dash pepper

2 or 3 tablespoons butter

15-ounce can tomato sauce (check for the
    lowest carbs and no added sugar)
1 clove garlic, minced
½ teaspoon onion powder
¼ teaspoon basil
⅛ teaspoon oregano

1. Combine the beef, Parmesan cheese, eggs parsley and pepper in mixer with a paddle beater on the lowest setting for 10 seconds.
1. Shape into forty 1-inch meatballs.
2. Melt the butter in a large skillet and cook the meatballs until all sides are browned. Remove to a Crock Pot or a casserole dish suitable for the oven.
3. Combine the tomato sauce, garlic, onion powder, basil, and oregano. Pour over the meatballs, gently stirring to coat.
4. Turn the Crock-Pot on low for 1 to 4 hours OR bake, uncovered, in an oven at 350° for 30 to 40 minutes—or until bubbly.

OPTIONS

• Although the butter adds a delicious flavor, instead of frying the meat balls you can place them on a large broiler tray plus rack and bake them at 350° for 10 minutes. Remove from oven, turn the meatballs upside down, and return to the oven for another 10 minutes.

These meatballs are great as a main dish or as an appetizer.

Tangy Meat Balls

2 pounds ground beef
2 eggs
1 cup finely chopped onion
1 tablespoon minced fresh parsley
1½ teaspoons ground coriander
1 teaspoon very finely chopped gingerroot
1 teaspoon chili powder
1 teaspoon paprika
1 teaspoon lemon-pepper spice blend
1 teaspoon salt

15-ounce can tomato sauce
1 cup finely chopped onion
1 clove garlic, minced
2 teaspoons paprika
1 teaspoon purchased spaghetti spice seasoning blend
1 teaspoon chili powder
1 teaspoon finely chopped gingerroot
¾ teaspoon ground coriander

1. Preheat oven to 350°.
2. Combine the beef, eggs, onion, parsley, coriander, gingerroot, chili powder, paprika, lemon-pepper, and salt in a mixer with the paddle on lowest setting for 10 seconds OR mix together by hand until just blended. Do not overmix.
3. Coat a broiler rack with vegetable oil spray. Shape the meat mixture into 3 dozen meatballs about 1½ inches in diameter. Place the meatballs on broiler rack. Bake for 10 minutes. Remove from the oven, turn the meatballs upside down, and bake for another 10 minutes.
4. Combine the tomato sauce, onion, garlic, paprika, spaghetti sauce seasoning, chili powder, gingerroot, and coriander. Stir in the baked meatballs, heat thoroughly and serve.

OPTIONS
- The meatballs can be browned on all sides in a large skillet in butter, but I find that baking them is faster and easier and they just fit on a regular-sized broiler rack.
- The meatballs and sauce can be cooked on low in a Crock-Pot.

These meatballs are spicy but not hot. This recipe has a delightfully unique flavor—something different from the more usual Italian or Swedish meat balls. Serve as a main course or as an appetizer.

Salisbury Steak

1 pound ground beef
1 egg
2 tablespoons finely diced green pepper
  (optional)
2 tablespoons finely diced onion
1 tablespoon minced fresh parsley
¼ teaspoon salt
Dash black pepper

1 tablespoon butter

½ cup cream
1 teaspoon Dijon mustard
1 teaspoon Worcestershire sauce
½ teaspoon horseradish

1. Combine the beef, egg, green pepper, onion, parsley, salt, and pepper in a mixer with the paddle on the lowest setting for 10 seconds OR mix together by hand until just blended. Do not overmix.
2. Shape the meat into a ball, then divide into fourths for quicker cooking. Shape into balls and flatten into 3-inch patties.
3. Melt the butter in a skillet. Place the patties in butter and cook to desired doneness, turning once or twice.
4. Combine the cream, mustard, Worcestershire sauce and horseradish and pour into the skillet. Simmer until thickened.
5. Serve the meat with the sauce poured over. Garnish with parsley, if desired.

> **This recipe makes 4 quarter-pounders. You can double this recipe to make 4 half-pound 'steaks.'**

Cottage Cheese and Hamburger Casserole

LOW CARBOHYDRATES   **NUMBER OF SERVINGS: 5 OR 6**

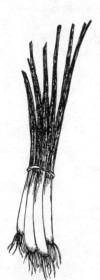

2 tablespoons butter
2 pounds ground beef

1 cup cottage cheese
½ cup sour cream
½ cup tomato paste
¼ teaspoon garlic powder
⅛ teaspoon black pepper
6 green onions, chopped, including tops
1 cup shredded cheddar cheese.

1. Preheat a broiler or convection broiler to high.
2. Melt the butter in an ovenproof skillet and add the beef. Cook on medium, stirring often, until browned and crumbled.
3. Add the cottage cheese, sour cream, tomato paste, garlic powder, and black pepper; heat through. Add the onions, then top with the cheese.
4. Broil or convection broil on high until the cheese is melted and slightly browned.

Green onions are a snap to grow. They can be planted very early in the spring, while the weather is still too cool for most crops. Purchase onion sets or seedlings, plant, and you can begin to harvest the green onions in less than a month!

Quick Creamed Hamburger and Mushrooms

VERY LOW CARBOHYDRATES   **NUMBER OF SERVINGS: 2 OR 3**

1 tablespoon butter
1 pound ground beef

4 ounces sliced fresh mushrooms
Dash of nutmeg
Dehydrated onion, one or two shakes, as desired
¼ teaspoon salt
⅛ teaspoon black pepper

32   *Back to Protein*

½ **cup heavy cream**

**Shredded cheese, cheddar/provolone blend
or as desired**

1. Melt the butter in a skillet, then brown and crumble the meat.
2. When the meat is nearly cooked, add the mushrooms, nutmeg, onion, salt, and pepper. Stir fry, mixing well, until the meat is done.
3. Add the cream and simmer briefly until thickened.
4. Serve topped with shredded cheese.

It's easy to double or triple this recipe. Leftovers heat well in the microwave.

Quick Creamed Hamburger and Onions

VERY LOW CARBOHYDRATES   **NUMBER OF SERVINGS: 2 OR 3**

1 tablespoon butter
1 pound ground beef

¼ *cup chopped onion*
¾ *teaspoon thyme*
¼ *teaspoon salt*
⅛ *teaspoon black pepper*

½ *cup heavy cream*

*Shredded cheese, cheddar/provolone blend
or as desired*

1. Melt the butter in skillet, then brown and crumble the meat.
2. When the meat is nearly cooked, add the onion, thyme, salt, and pepper. Stir fry, mixing well, until meat is done.
3. Add the cream and simmer briefly until thickened.
4. Serve topped with shredded cheese.

It's easy to double or triple this recipe. Leftovers heat well in the microwave.

"Sloppy Joes" in Barbecue Sauce

VERY LOW CARBOHYDRATES   **NUMBER OF SERVINGS: 2 OR 3**

1 tablespoon butter or olive oil
1 pound ground beef

⅓ cup water
¼ cup Westbrae Unsweetened Un-Ketchup
1 tablespoon dried minced onion
1 teaspoon prepared mustard
1 teaspoon prepared horseradish
1 teaspoon Worcestershire
Dash black pepper

1. Melt the butter in a skillet; add the beef. Brown the beef on medium, stirring to crumble.
2. Add the water, Un-Ketchup, onion, mustard, horseradish, Worcestershire sauce, and black pepper. Simmer until the liquid evaporates and the sauce is somewhat thick.

> This tastes just like the canned sloppy joe barbecue sauce you add to hamburger—only without the sugar!

Mock Cheeseburgers

TRACE OF CARBOHYDRATES   **NUMBER OF SERVINGS: 2 OR 3**

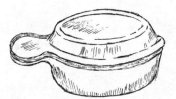

1 tablespoon olive oil
1 pound ground beef

Shredded cheddar or cheddar-blend cheeses
4 slices bacon, cooked crisp

1. Brown and crumble meat in skillet with olive oil. Divide into individual serving dishes.
2. Top each with a generous portion of shredded cheese and 2 crisp slices of bacon.

OPTIONS

• To save time, brown at least 2 or 3 pounds of ground beef, place the meat in individual containers (I use Corelle serving dishes), top each with a generous serving of cheese and freeze or refrigerate. When ready to eat, cook some bacon in the microwave or on the stove, heat up the hamburger and cheese in the microwave on high for about one minute. Then top with the bacon and serve.

• Consider using inexpensive paper bowls for individual containers—they go well in the refrigerator and microwave. To freeze, seal in plastic.

This is one of my favorites for breakfast!

Berneice's Hamburger and Chipped Beef Roll-ups

LOW CARBOHYDRATES   **NUMBER OF SERVINGS: 2**

1 pound ground beef
1 egg (optional)
Salt and pepper as desired

1 to 2 ounces thinly sliced cooked beef
½ cup shredded mozzarella cheese

1. Preheat the oven or convection oven to 350°.
2. Mix the ground beef, egg, salt, and pepper. Flatten the mixture on waxed paper to about 8½ inches square.
3. Place the thinly sliced cooked beef in layers over the hamburger. Sprinkle with cheese.
4. Roll the meat into a log, peeling back the waxed paper as you go. Press the ends to seal in the cheese. Place in a bread loaf pan.
5. Bake for 45 minutes or convection bake for 30 minutes or until done. Slice and serve.

OPTIONS

• Instead of mozzarella, substitute 2 ounces of Philadelphia cream cheese brought to room temperature so you can easily spread it over the beef. Roll up and bake as above.
• Other variations include: sprinkle on a few capers, black olive slices, green pepper strips, pepperoni, or sliced green olives stuffed with pimento.

Quick Hamburger-Green Pepper Skillet

VERY LOW CARBOHYDRATES   **NUMBER OF SERVINGS: 2**

> 1 tablespoon butter
> 1 pound ground beef
> ¼ green pepper, cut into strips OR chopped onion OR a combination
> Mozzarella-provolone mix, shredded

1. Melt butter in a skillet on medium heat. Cook and crumble ground beef.
2. Add the green pepper. Stir-fry until the pepper is tender and beef is browned.
3. Top with shredded cheese and serve.

OPTIONS

- One minced garlic clove can be added with the green pepper.
- One medium tomato, cut into chunks, can be added with the green pepper.
- Meat can be topped with a little shredded mozzarella cheese.
- All three previous options can be combined together—it's great!

Bob likes the main recipe with a little low-carb salsa.

Hamburger with Whipped Cream and Horseradish

VERY LOW CARBOHYDRATES   **NUMBER OF SERVINGS: 2**

> 1 tablespoon butter
> 1 pound ground beef
>
> Shredded cheddar or cheese of choice
>
> ½ cup heavy whipping cream, whipped till stiff
> 2 to 3 tablespoons prepared horseradish

1. Melt the butter in a skillet; brown and crumble ground beef. Top with cheese.
2. Combine whipped cream and horseradish. Put a dollop on each serving.

OPTIONS

- The meat can be pattied and fried or grilled, then topped with a slice of cheese and a dollop of whipped cream and horseradish.
- The whipped cream and horseradish tastes great on meat—even without the cheese.

Leftovers are great reheated in the microwave. Heat the meat and the cheese but not the whipped cream and horseradish, which should be added after the hamburger is hot.

Beef and Almond Casserole

LOW CARBOHYDRATES   NUMBER OF SERVINGS: 4 OR 5

> 2 tablespoons butter
> 2 pounds ground beef
>
> ½ cup chopped celery
> ¼ cup chopped green pepper
> ¼ cup chopped onion
> 2-ounce jar sliced pimento, drained
> 4 to 6 fresh mushrooms, sliced OR a 4-ounce can of sliced mushrooms, drained
>
> 2 to 4 tablespoons soy sauce
> Up to 1 cup sour cream
>
> ⅓ cup sliced almonds, toasted a few seconds under broiler

1. Melt the butter in a skillet. Brown and crumble ground beef.
2. Add the celery, green pepper, onion, pimento, and mushrooms. Stir-fry 2 or 3 minutes.
3. Add the soy sauce and sour cream, stirring well. Heat through, but do not boil.
4. Top with the toasted almonds and serve.

Beef and Green Bean Casserole

LOW CARBOHYDRATES   NUMBER OF SERVINGS: 5

1 to 2 tablespoons olive oil or butter
2 pounds ground beef

4-ounce can sliced mushrooms, drained
14.5-ounce can French-style green beans, drained
1 teaspoon Worcestershire sauce (optional)
Salt and pepper to taste

1 to 1½ cups heavy cream
1 to 1½ cup shredded cheddar cheese (or other cheese)

Crumbled pork rinds

1. Preheat broiler to high.
2. Cook and crumble the ground beef in the oil in an ovenproof skillet on medium heat.
3. Add the mushrooms, beans, Worcestershire sauce, salt, and pepper. Stir together and heat through.
4. Add the cream and simmer until thickened.
5. Top with the shredded cheese. Place under the broiler a few seconds until the cheese is melted and lightly browned.
6. Remove from the broiler, top with crumbled pork rinds, and serve.

OPTIONS
- Substitute lightly toasted almond slivers for the crumbled pork rinds.

Chili without Beans

LOW CARBOHYDRATES   NUMBER OF SERVINGS: 2

1 tablespoon butter
1 pound ground beef
⅓ cup chopped onion

8-ounce can tomato sauce (check that no sugar has been added)
½ teaspoon beef bouillon granules
½ to 1 teaspoon chili powder, or more to taste

Shredded cheddar cheese
Sour cream

1 .Melt the butter in a skillet. Brown the beef and onion together.
2. Add the tomato sauce, beef bouillon granules, and chili powder. Simmer together 2 or 3 minutes.
3. Serve in individual bowls. Top with cheddar cheese and a dollop of sour cream.

Coconut Beef Curry

LOW CARBOHYDRATES   **NUMBER OF SERVINGS: 2**

1 tablespoon olive oil
1 pound ground beef
⅓ cup chopped onion

1 cup beef broth
⅓ cup flaked coconut (the kind with no sugar added)
1 teaspoon curry powder
1 teaspoon garlic powder
¼ teaspoon cinnamon

2 tablespoons pecan pieces, coarsely chopped

1. Brown and crumble the beef and onions in olive oil in a skillet on medium high heat.
2. Add the broth, coconut, curry, garlic, and cinnamon. Simmer together until the broth is nearly gone.
3. Serve topped with pecan pieces.

OPTIONS
- Although this delicious recipe qualifies as low carb, reduce the carbs even more by cutting the onion and coconut back to ¼ cup and eliminate the pecans.
- If you like hotter food, increase the curry and garlic to 1 ½ or 2 teaspoons each and the cinnamon to ½ teaspoon.

I tried to emulate the spice flavors from an Indian cooking class I took years ago. The dish was served with silver leaf on top, giving the nuts a sheen that was quite attractive.

Beef and Pepperoni "Pizza"

LOW CARBOHYDRATES: **NUMBER OF SERVINGS: 6**

2 tablespoons olive oil
2 pounds ground beef

3 to 4 cups low-carb tomato sauce
3 teaspoons purchased pizza spice blend
Garlic powder as desired
Purchased Pizza peppers blend as desired
8 ounces pepperoni, cut into slivers
¾ cup chopped onion
6 tablespoons green pepper, chopped
4 ounce can sliced mushrooms, drained
12 black olives, sliced
6 tablespoons grated Parmesan cheese
2½ to 3 cups finely shredded mozzarella
    cheese

1. Preheat oven to 400°.
2. Brown and crumble the beef in the olive oil in a skillet.
3. Divide the remaining ingredients among 6 serving dishes—I use
   Corning oval individual servers that measure 4½ by 7¼ inches. Place
   the following in each dish, in the order given:

¼ to ⅓ cup tomato sauce, spread to cover
    the bottom
⅓ pound browned beef
½ teaspoon pizza spice blend
Dash garlic powder and pizza peppers, in
    amounts desired
Just over 1 ounce of the pepperoni slivers
2 tablespoons chopped onion
1 tablespoon chopped green pepper
⅙ of the canned mushrooms
2 black olives, sliced
¼ to ⅓ cup additional tomato sauce
1 or 2 tablespoons grated Parmesan cheese
⅓ to ½ cup mozzarella cheese

4. Place the individual serving dishes on a jellyroll pan or cookie sheet
   and bake in the oven for 15 minutes or in a convection for about 10
   minutes—or until bubbly and the cheese is lightly browned. Serve on
   charger plates or hot pads.

• Any of the toppings can be reduced or eliminated. If you put in the maximum amounts listed, the carb counts are over 12 grams per serving.

• **Each serving is a meal in itself, and it all goes together faster than you might think!**
• **This dish freezes well. Just cover each serving dish carefully; the Corning dishes I use come with wonderful plastic snap-on lids. This dish also reheats very well in the microwave.**

Bacon, Beef and Sausage "Pizza"

LOW CARBOHYDRATES   **NUMBER OF SERVINGS: 3**

¼ pound bacon
½ pound ground beef
½ pound seasoned bulk sausage

8-ounce can tomato sauce
Dash garlic powder, perhaps ⅛ teaspoon total
¾ teaspoon oregano
4 ounces sliced canned mushrooms, drained
1½ to 2¼ cups shredded mozzarella/provolone cheese blend

1. Preheat the oven to 375°.
2. Cook the bacon in a large skillet until crisp. Drain the strips on a paper towel. Pour off the fat remaining in the skillet.
3. Cook the ground beef and sausage together in the skillet, crumbling and stirring until browned. Drain off the liquid and fat.
4. Stir garlic powder and oregano into the tomato sauce. Divide the tomato sauce among 3 individual serving dishes—I use Corning French white ovals.
5. Top the tomato sauce first with the bacon, and then with the beef and sausage mixture.
6. Place the mushrooms on top of the meat and then top each serving dish with ½ to ¾ cup mozzarella/provolone cheese blend.
7. Place on a cookie sheet and bake in the oven for 20 minutes—or until the cheeses are lightly browned.

This "pizza" is ready to eat in less than 40 minutes.

Taco Salad

1 tablespoon olive oil
1 pound ground beef
½ cup chopped onion

4 teaspoons Homemade Taco Seasoning Mix
(see below)
⅓ cup water

Lettuce
Sour cream
Chopped green onions
Shredded cheddar cheese
Black olives, sliced
Chopped tomato
Salsa (check that it's low-carb)

1. In a skillet, brown and crumble the beef and onions in the oil.
2. Prepare the Homemade Taco Seasoning Mix. Combine the following:

4 tablespoons chili powder (can increase, to
taste)
1 tablespoon garlic powder
1 tablespoon cumin
1½ teaspoons salt, or to taste

Store in a jar for future use.

3. Add 4 teaspoons of the taco seasoning mix and the water. Stir well. Simmer until the water has boiled away.
4. Serve the meat mixture on a bed of lettuce topped with a dollop of sour cream, green onions, cheddar cheese, black olives, and chopped tomato. Pass the salsa!

OPTIONS
• The lettuce or any of the toppings can be eliminated if desired.

This is a speedy recipe and the Homemade Taco Seasoning Mix tastes just like the prepackaged taco mix—without the carbs and preservatives!

Chili Salad

1 tablespoon olive oil
2 pounds ground beef
1 medium onion, chopped
1 small green pepper, chopped

14.5-ounce can whole tomatoes in tomato
    juice (12 grams total)
¼ cup Westbrae Unsweetened Un-Ketchup
1 tablespoon chili powder
2 tablespoons purchased Italian spice blend
1½ teaspoons celery salt
1 tablespoon black pepper
1 teaspoon garlic powder

Lettuce of choice
1 cup shredded cheddar cheese

1. Cook the beef, onion, and green pepper in the oil in a skillet until the meat is browned and crumbled.
2. Add all of the remaining ingredients except the lettuce and cheese; simmer for about 5 minutes or until thickened.
3. Spoon the meat mixture over the lettuce and top with cheese.

OPTIONS
• The chili powder and black pepper can be doubled, if a hotter chili is desired.

My Great Mock Lasagna

3 tablespoons butter or olive oil
3 pounds ground beef

2 tablespoons butter or olive oil
6 ounces fresh mushrooms

1 green pepper
1 large onion
½ cup black olives, sliced
15 ounce can tomato sauce
12 ounce can tomato paste
1 tablespoon purchased Italian spice blend
   (or more, if desired)
Scant ½ teaspoon fennel seeds
2 teaspoons dried basil OR ¼ cup fresh,
   chopped basil
1 tablespoon chicken bouillon granules
1 teaspoon thyme OR 1 tablespoons fresh,
   chopped thyme
3 large cloves garlic, minced
¼ teaspoon black pepper
Salt to taste (optional)

24-ounce carton cottage cheese, about 3
   cups, drained
2 egg yolks
1 tablespoon dried parsley OR 3 tablespoons fresh, minced parsley

12 ounces (or more) shredded mozzarella
   cheese
¾ cup grated Parmesan cheese

1. Preheat the oven to 400°. Set out 3 mixing bowls.
2. Place the 3 tablespoons of butter or oil in a large skillet. Add the ground beef and cook on medium, browning and crumbling the meat.
3. While the meat is cooking, put the 2 tablespoons of butter or oil in a medium skillet and cook the mushrooms on medium heat, stirring occasionally.
4. Run the green pepper, and onion olives through a food processor using the smallest slicing blade OR chop by hand. Place the chopped pepper, onion, and olives in the largest mixing bowl, along

with the tomato sauce, paste, Italian spice blend, fennel seeds, basil, chicken bouillon, thyme, garlic, pepper, and salt.

5. When the meat and mushrooms are cooked, combine with the tomato sauce mixture. This is bowl one.
6. In bowl two, combine the cottage cheese, egg yolks, and parsley.
7. In bowl three, combine the mozzarella and Parmesan cheese.

To assemble the lasagna:

8. Spray a large lasagna pan, 11½ by 16 inches, OR two smaller pans with vegetable oil.
9. Layer half the ingredients from each bowl in the lasagna pan, in the order given, starting with bowl 1, then bowl 2, and bowl 3. Repeat.
10. Cover the lasagna with foil and bake for 25 minutes. Remove the cover and bake another 25 minutes—or until bubbly and the cheese is browned. Cut and serve.

OPTIONS

• Although you can halve this recipe, I usually make the full batch to fit in my large lasagna pan and reheat leftovers in the microwave.

This low-carb lasagna was adapted from my original high-carb recipe, which called for my homemade pasta and tomato sauce created from produce grown in my garden. Once my husband conned me into making an extra batch and freezing it for my own surprise birthday party!

CROCK POT SAFETY

The following recipes can be cooked in a Crock-Pot. The Iowa State University Extension offers the following safety tips:

TO DETERMINE IF A SLOW COOKER WILL HEAT FOOD TO A SAFE TEMPERATURE:

1. Fill the cooker with 2 quarts of water.
2. Heat on Low for 8 hours or to the desired cooking time.
3. Check the water temperature with an accurate thermometer (do this quickly because the temperature drops 10 to 15 degrees when the lid is removed).
4. The temperature of the water should be 185° to 200° F. Temperatures above this would indicate that a product cooked for 8 hours without stirring would be overdone. Temperatures below this may indicate the cooker does not heat food high enough or fast enough to avoid potential food safety problems.

WHEN USING A SLOW COOKER, FOLLOW THESE GUIDELINES:

1. Start with fresh or thawed meat—not frozen.
2. Use chunks rather than large cuts or roasts. Use pieces of poultry—not a whole chicken.
3. Cook meat on high for 1 hour and then turn the cooker to low rather than cook on low for the entire length of time.
4. Only use recipes that include a liquid.
5. Use a thermometer to check the internal temperature to make sure food reaches 160° F.
6. Do not delay starting time.
7. Do not reheat foods in slow cooker.
8. Keep the lid on.

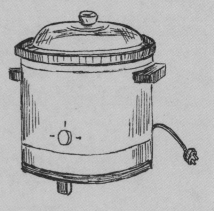

Back to Protein

Basic Beef Stew

2 pounds lean beef stew meat, cubed
4 ribs celery, cut into 1 inch chunks
1 small carrot or ½ large one, cut into ½
   inch chunks
1 large onion, chopped
2 14-ounce cans whole tomatoes,
   undrained, but check for added sugar
1 teaspoon beef bouillon granules
⅛ teaspoon pepper
1 teaspoon basil
2 cloves garlic, minced

1. Place all of the ingredients in a Crock-Pot all day on low. Serve in bowls.
2. Place all of the ingredients in a covered OR oven-proof pan and bake
   at 325° for 2½ to 3 hours.

OPTIONS
• Brown the beef in a skillet with a little olive oil, if you prefer, before putting it in the Crock-Pot.

My butcher provides me with wonderful extra lean stew meat already
cubed. But you can substitute a beef roast or cheap cut of steak and cut the
cubes yourself, trimming off any excess fat.

Beef & Beer Stew

VERY LOW CARBOHYDRATES   **NUMBER OF SERVINGS: 5 OR 6**

2 tablespoons olive oil
2½ pounds lean beef stew meat, cubed
2 medium onions, sliced

1 can Miller Lite Beer
½ teaspoon thyme
1 tablespoon Westbrae Unsweetened Un-Ketchup
1 teaspoon soy sauce
1 teaspoon Worcestershire sauce
1 garlic clove, minced
1 bay leaf

1. In a large skillet, brown the meat and onions in the olive oil. If time is short, you can eliminate this step.
2. Mix the remaining ingredients in a crock pot. Stir in the onions and meat. Cover and cook on low all day or on high for half a day. Serve in bowls.

OPTIONS

• If you had bacon for breakfast, drain the excess grease out of the skillet (without scraping) and use this to cook the meat and bacon, omitting the olive oil. Delicious!

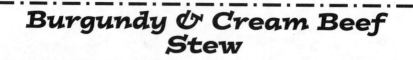

This recipe takes just moments to make in the morning. It can cook all day while you're at work and, when you come home, supper is ready!

Burgundy & Cream Beef Stew

LOW CARBOHYDRATES   **NUMBER OF SERVINGS: 5 OR 6**

4 tablespoons butter
2½ pounds lean beef stew meat, cubed
2 onions, thinly sliced
1 clove garlic, minced

2 cups beef broth (14- ounce can)
½ cup burgundy cooking wine
¼ teaspoon marjoram
¼ teaspoon oregano
¼ teaspoon black pepper
¼ teaspoon salt

½ cup sour cream plus more for garnish
Parsley sprigs for garnish (optional)

1. Melt the butter in a large skillet and add the meat, onions, and garlic. Brown together. This step is optional, if time is short.
2. In a Crock-Pot, mix together the broth, wine, marjoram, oregano, black pepper, and salt. Stir in the meat and onions. Cover and cook on low all day or on high for half a day.
3. Fifteen minutes before serving, stir in ½ cup sour cream. Serve in bowls with a small dollop of sour cream on top, garnished with a sprig of parsley.

OPTIONS

• If you had bacon for breakfast, drain the excess grease out of the skillet (without scraping) and use this to cook the meat and bacon, omitting the olive oil. Delicious!

Burgundy Beef Stew

LOW CARBOHYDRATES   **NUMBER OF SERVINGS: 6**

2½ pounds lean beef stew meat, cubed
2 cups beef broth (homemade or canned)
1 cup burgundy wine
8 ounces mushrooms, sliced
1 coarsely chopped green pepper
1 medium onion, chopped
3 or 4 ribs celery, sliced (about 1 cup)
1 teaspoon salt

1. Stir all of the ingredients together in a Crock-Pot. Cover and cook on low all day or on high for half a day. Serve in bowls.
OR Bake in the oven, covered, at 400° until it starts to bubble, reduce the heat to 250° for 3 or 4 hours.
OR Bring to a boil in a heavy saucepan on the stove, then reduce the heat and simmer for half a day, stirring occasionally. Do not leave the stove unattended for hours.

OPTIONS

• Brown the beef in a little olive oil before putting it in the Crock-Pot, if you like.

Cabbage Beef Stew

LOW OR VERY LOW CARBOHYDRATES   **NUMBER OF SERVINGS: 2 OR 3**

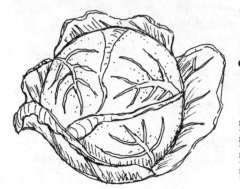

1 pound lean beef stew
    meat, cubed
1½ cups coarsely chopped
cabbage
1 onion, coarsely chopped
14 ounce can beef broth
1 bay leaf
¼ teaspoon salt or as desired
¼ pepper or as desired
⅛ teaspoon sage
⅛ teaspoon rosemary

Stir all of the ingredients together in the Crock-Pot. Cook, covered, all day on low or half a day on high. Remove the bay leaf when serving.

OPTIONS
• You can brown the beef in a little olive oil before putting it in the Crock-Pot, if you like.
• This recipe can easily be doubled.

Cashew Stew

LOW CARBOHYDRATES   **NUMBER OF SERVINGS: 3**

1 pound lean beef stew meat, cubed
1 medium onion, coarsely chopped
¾ cup chopped celery (3 outer ribs)
4 ounce can sliced mushrooms, including
    liquid
½ cup whole cashews
¼ teaspoon salt or to taste

Stir all of the ingredients together in the Crock-Pot. Cook, covered, all day on low or half a day on high. Serve in bowls.

OPTIONS
• You can brown the beef in a little olive oil before putting it in the Crock-Pot, if you like.
• This recipe can easily be doubled.

Lemon Beef Stew

LOW CARBOHYDRATES   **NUMBER OF SERVINGS: 6 TO 8**

About 3 pounds lean beef stew meat, cubed
2 medium onions, coarsely chopped
1 cup tomato sauce
1 small carrot, chopped
1 small unpeeled lemon, washed and thinly
*   sliced; discard ends and seeds*
1 tablespoon Worcestershire sauce
½ teaspoon salt
¼ teaspoon pepper

1. Combine all of the ingredients in a Crock-Pot. Cover and cook all
   day on low or half a day on high.
OR Combine all of the ingredients and bake in the oven at 300° for 3 or
   4 hours or until the meat is tender.

OPTIONS

• Add ½ a green pepper, chopped.
• Add mushrooms, canned or fresh, as desired.

**The lemon slices can be eaten OR you can cook the stew with
the lemons on top and pick them out before serving.**

Spanish Beef Stew

VERY LOW CARBOHYDRATES   **NUMBER OF SERVINGS: 4 OR 5**

2 pounds lean beef stew meat, cubed
4-ounce jar sliced red pimentos, undrained
1 large clove garlic, peeled
1 bay leaf
¼ teaspoon black pepper
½ cup water
1 teaspoon concentrated beef broth or
1 teaspoon granulated beef bouillon

1. Combine ingredients in crock pot, cover, and cook all day on low or
   half a day on high.
2. Serve in bowls with the broth.

OPTIONS

• Brown the beef in a heavy saucepan in a little butter. Add the other ingredients and simmer
  on low until the meat is tender, about 2 hours.
• Bake in the oven at 350° in a tightly covered casserole dish for 1 or 2 hours.

Beef   **51**

Tomato & Pepper Beef Stew

LOW CARBOHYDRATES

NUMBER OF SERVINGS: 5 OR 6

2½ pounds lean beef stew meat, cubed OR
    round bottom boneless roast
2 tablespoons butter

1 pound can tomatoes in juice
1 large onion, cut into bite-sized chunks
1 green pepper, cut into bite-sized chunks
1 large clove garlic, minced
Salt and pepper as desired

1. Melt the butter in a large skillet and brown the beef on all sides.
2. Add the remaining ingredients. Simmer on low an hour or more until meat is tender and vegetables are tender but not mushy.

Tomato & Mushroom Stew

LOW CARBOHYDRATES

NUMBER OF SERVINGS: 10

About 5½ pounds arm roast, trimmed of
    excess fat and cut into 1-inch cubes OR
    lean beef stew meat
28-ounce can crushed tomatoes
1 cup burgundy wine
1 tablespoon beef bouillon granules
8 ounces mushrooms, sliced

1. Combine ingredients in covered Crock-Pot cooking on high all day. Serve.

OPTIONS

• If desired, brown the meat in 3 tablespoons of butter or olive oil in a skillet before adding to the Crock-Pot.

> If you halve the recipe, you can cook it in a Crock-Pot on low all day or on high for half a day.

Mock Beef Stroganoff Stew

2 tablespoons butter
1 large onion, sliced
1 large clove garlic, peeled and diced

1 to 2 tablespoons butter
3 pounds lean beef stew meat, cubed OR
top round steak cut into strips

8 ounces mushrooms, sliced
1 teaspoon black pepper

1 cup burgundy cooking wine
½ cup Westbrae Unsweetened Un-Ketchup
½ cup sour cream (optional) plus additional
for topping (optional)

1. Melt the butter in a skillet and cook the onions and garlic until brown and tender on medium heat, about 5 minutes. Place in Crock-Pot, oven casserole, or stew pot.
2. Melt the additional butter in the skillet and add the meat, stirring to brown all sides, for about 5 minutes. Add the mushrooms and black pepper and cook another 5 minutes. Stir into the onions.
3. Cook in a covered crock pot all day on low, or half a day on high. Bake, covered at 275° for 3 or 4 hours or until the meat is tender.
OR Simmer, covered, in a heavy saucepan on the stove for an hour or two or until the meat is tender.
4. Add the burgundy, Un-ketchup, and ½ cup sour cream; heat through. Serve topped with a dollop of sour cream.

Mock Chimichangas

2 pounds lean beef stew meat, cubed
⅔ cup water OR beef broth
2 cloves garlic, minced
1 tablespoon chili powder
1 tablespoon vinegar
2 teaspoons oregano
1 teaspoon cumin
½ teaspoon salt
Dash pepper

Lettuce
Sour cream
Shredded cheddar cheese
Diced green onion, including tops, OR
chopped chives

1. Place the meat, water, or beef broth, garlic, chili powder, vinegar, oregano, cumin, salt and pepper in covered Crock-Pot all day on low or half a day on high OR simmer, covered, in a heavy sauce pan for 2 or 3 hours or until the meat is tender—checking that the liquid doesn't evaporate.
2. Using two forks, shred the meat. The remaining liquid should be absorbed into the shredded meat; if not, simmer a little longer until it's nearly gone.
3. Serve on a bed of lettuce topped with sour cream, shredded cheddar, and green onion.

OPTIONS
• Serve with a little guacamole and garnish with tomato slices.
• Top with a little low-carb salsa and sliced black olives.

This is truly outstanding—and you don't miss the tortillas!

Sour Cream Beef in Crock Pot

2 tablespoons butter or olive oil
2 pounds lean beef stew meat, cubed
1 large onion, sliced

½ cup sour cream
¼ cup shredded cheddar cheese
Salt and pepper to taste

1. Melt the butter in a large skillet and brown the beef and onions.
2. Combine the beef and onions, sour cream, cheddar cheese, salt and pepper in a Crock-Pot. Cover and cook all day on low. Do NOT cook half a day on high because the sour cream will separate.

OPTIONS

• Add some sliced or canned mushrooms and cook them in the butter with the meat and onions.
• Omit the salt and add 8 to 12 sliced black olives to the dish before serving. Do NOT cook the olives in the Crock-Pot because it will make the meat taste too salty.

Basic Beef Roast

NO CARBOHYDRATES   **NUMBER OF SERVINGS: AS DESIRED**

One beef rump roast, allow at least ½
pound per serving
Water
Garlic powder (optional)
Salt and pepper as desired

1. Preheat oven to 350° or 400° on bake. Coat a roasting pan with vegetable oil spray. Place the roast in the pan, then bake for 15 to 30 minutes, uncovered, to brown the outside of the meat.
2. Sprinkle the roast with garlic powder, salt, and pepper as desired. Pour a little water into the bottom of the roaster, to a depth of 1/4 inch or so. Cover and bake until the meat is at the desired doneness, turning the meat or basting from time to time, adding more water if necessary. Slice and serve.

OPTIONS

• Pour pan juices into a bowl and skim off the fat with a spoon OR use a separator. Spoon the remaining broth over slices of the roast—delicious!
• After the meat has browned, coat the top of the roast with Kitchen Bouquet, if desired, which enriches the flavor of both the meat and the juices.

• **Allow roast to rest, covered, on the counter for 10 minutes before slicing, and it will cut neatly.**
• **Leftover meat is great eaten cold, heated in the microwave, or cut up and added to a lettuce salad.**

Beef Roast with a Hint of Barbecue Flavor

VERY LOW CARBOHYDRATES   **NUMBER OF SERVINGS: 4 OR 5**

> 3 tablespoons red wine vinegar
> 3 tablespoons Westbrae Unsweetened Un-Ketchup
> 2 tablespoons Worcestershire sauce
> 2 tablespoons soy sauce
> ½ teaspoon dried rosemary, crushed in a mortar and pestle
> ½ teaspoon garlic powder
> ½ teaspoon dry mustard
>
> 2 pound beef roast

1. Preheat the oven to 350°.
2. Combine all of the ingredients except the meat in a bowl to make the sauce.
3. Coat a small roasting pan or covered casserole dish with vegetable oil spray. Add the meat and pour the sauce over the roast. Cover and bake to desired doneness. Allow to rest on the counter for 10 minutes, covered, then slice and serve with pan juices spooned over meat.

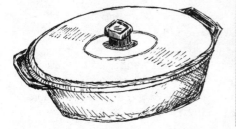

Cold leftovers make a great salad. Cut the meat into bite-sized chunks and place on a bed of lettuce with a little chopped celery. Top the salad with the pan juices, which become liquid at room temperature and make a great dressing.

Beef Roast with Horseradish

VERY LOW CARBOHYDRATES   **NUMBER OF SERVINGS: 4 OR 5**

> 2 pounds beef roast
> 2 garlic cloves, minced
> ⅓ cup prepared horseradish OR to taste
> 1 large onion, sliced
> ½ cup water or amount needed to coat the bottom of roaster

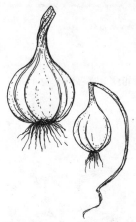

1. Preheat the oven to 350°.
2. Coat a roasting pan with vegetable oil spray. Place the meat in the roaster.
3. Rub the garlic into the top of the roast.
4. Spread the horseradish on top of the roast.
5. Lay the onion slices over the roast.
6. Pour the water in the bottom of the pan.
7. Cover and bake until the meat is at the desired doneness, basting from time to time with pan juices or adding more water if necessary.
8. Allow to rest on the counter for 10 minutes, covered, then slice and serve with pan juices spooned over the meat.

Beef Roast with Sauerkraut

LOW CARBOHYDRATES   **NUMBER OF SERVINGS: 5 OR 6**

One large onion, peeled and sliced
2½ to 3-pound beef roast
2 strips bacon
14 ounce can sauerkraut, undrained
1 cup hot water
Salt and pepper to taste
Caraway seeds, if desired

1. Preheat the oven to 350°.
2. Place the onion slices in a layer on the bottom of a covered roasting pan or casserole dish. Top with the roast.
3. Lay 2 strips of bacon over the meat.
3. Pour the sauerkraut and water over the meat. Sprinkle with salt and pepper and a dash of caraway seeds, to taste.
4. Bake, covered, for 2 or 3 hours or to desired doneness.
5. Allow to rest on the counter for 10 minutes, covered, then slice and serve with pan juices and sauerkraut spooned over meat.

> **Bob hates sauerkraut but really likes this recipe.**

Ebb's Italian Wedding Beef Roast

VERY LOW CARBOHYDRATES **NUMBER OF SERVINGS: 4 OR 5**

2-pound beef roast
Dash salt

½ teaspoon garlic powder
½ teaspoon dried basil
  OR use fresh sprigs
  as desired
¼ cup grated Parmesan
  or Parmesan-
  Romano blend
  cheese
1 green pepper, thinly
  sliced in food
  processor using nar-
  rowest blades
14.5-ounce can beef
  broth

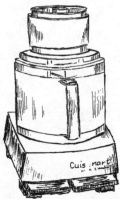

1. Place the beef in a pan. Sprinkle with salt. Bake, uncovered, at 325° for 1 hour. Let cool and slice thin.
2. Layer the meat, garlic powder, basil leaves, cheese, and green pepper in a pan with a tightly fitting lid. Repeat the layers. Pour the broth over all.
3. Bake, covered, at 325° for 2 or more hours to desired doneness. Baste once or twice as it bakes.
4. Serve with pan juices spooned over the meat.

> **Multiply this recipe as needed. It can be prepared in advance, then refrigerated or frozen and reheated it when desired.**

Roast Beef with Beer

VERY LOW CARBOHYDRATES **NUMBER OF SERVINGS: 7 OR 8**

4-pound beef roast
1 ½ cups chopped celery (about 3 ribs)
½ cup sliced carrot (1 medium)
1 large onion, quartered and sliced
Zest from 1 lemon
4-ounce can mushrooms, undrained

1 bay leaf
½ teaspoon salt OR 1 teaspoon beef bouillon granules

¼ teaspoon pepper
12-ounce can Miller Lite Beer

1. Preheat oven to 325° degrees.
2. Place the meat in a covered roasting pan or casserole. Top with the remaining ingredients.
3. Cover and bake 3 or 4 hours to desired doneness.
4. Allow to rest on the counter for 10 minutes, covered, then slice and serve with pan juices and spooned over meat.

OPTIONS
• After baking, cut the roast into chunks and return the meat to the liquid to create a stew or soup.
• Substitute 4 pounds of stew meat, cubed, and bake, simmer on the stovetop, or cook in a Crock-Pot on high all day. Wonderful!

This smells heavenly as it cooks!

Barbecued Beef Roast with Cola

VERY LOW CARBOHYDRATES   **NUMBER OF SERVINGS: 7 OR 8**

4 pound beef roast
2 cups no-carb cola beverage
8-ounce can tomato sauce
¼ cup vinegar
1 tablespoon dried minced onion
½ teaspoon celery seed
¼ teaspoon dry mustard
⅛ teaspoon cinnamon
⅛ teaspoon ground cloves

1. Preheat oven to 350°, (convection oven to 325°).
2. Place the roast in the bottom of a deep-sided roasting pan or casserole dish just large enough to hold the meat without it touching the sides.
3. Combine the remaining ingredients and pour over the meat. Bake, uncovered, 2 or 3 hours or almost to desired doneness, turning the meat once or twice.
4. When nearly done, slice the roast and return the meat to the liquid in the pan and bake, uncovered, 30 to 60 minutes. Serve.

OPTIONS
• This version is mild. If you prefer, double the dry spices for a stronger flavor.

Beef **59**

Be aware that no-carb cola contains artificial sweeteners. We have such strong misgivings about them that this is one of only two recipes in this book with artificial sweeteners. You may wish to avoid artificial sweeteners or consume them only occasionally. For another Barbecued Beef Roast without the artificial sweeteners, see the next recipe.

Barbecued Beef Roast

VERY LOW CARBOHYDRATES　　　　　　　　　　**NUMBER OF SERVINGS: 6 TO 8**

4- to 5-pound round bottom roast
¼ cup Liquid Smoke
2½ tablespoons celery seeds
2 tablespoons soy sauce
2½ tablespoons Worcestershire sauce
1½ tablespoons dried onion flakes
1 tablespoon dry minced garlic
1½ teaspoons black pepper

1. Place the roast in a large, durable plastic bag. Mix the rest of the ingredients in a bowl then pour over the meat. Seal the bag and store in the refrigerator overnight.
2. Preheat the oven to 325°.
3. Remove the roast and marinade from the plastic bag and put both in a covered roasting pan. Bake for 3 or 4 hours or until tender and to desired doneness, turning occasionally.
4. Let sit on the counter for 10 minutes, then slice and serve.

Marinated Beef Roast

VERY LOW CARBOHYDRATES   **NUMBER OF SERVINGS: 6 OR 7**

14-ounce can beef broth
⅓ cup soy sauce
¼ cup lemon juice
1 teaspoon Liquid Smoke
2 cloves garlic, minced
3-pound beef roast

1. Combine the broth, soy sauce, lemon juice, Liquid Smoke, and garlic.
2. Place the beef roast in a covered roasting pan or casserole large enough to hold the roast without it touching the sides. Pour the broth mixture over the roast and marinate overnight. Turn the roast once, if convenient.
3. Bake the roast with the marinade, covered, at 325° for 2 or 3 hours, or to desired doneness.
4. Allow to rest on the counter for 10 minutes, covered, then slice and serve with pan juices spooned over meat.

Roast Beef with Gingerroot

VERY LOW CARBOHYDRATES   **NUMBER OF SERVINGS: 6 TO 8**

3 pound bottom round roast

½ cup soy sauce
¼ cup sherry cooking wine
1 tablespoon minced gingerroot OR ½
    tablespoon dry ginger
1 clove garlic, minced

1. Place the roast in a large, durable plastic bag.
2. Combine the soy sauce, sherry, gingerroot and garlic. Mix with a hand blender to thoroughly blend the ingredients. Pour over the roast and seal the plastic bag.
3. Refrigerate for 2 hours or longer. Rotate occasionally.
4. Preheat an outdoor grill on high. Remove the roast from plastic bag and place on the grill. Close the lid and reduce the heat to medium-low. Turn the roast every 10 minutes. Cook to desired doneness, then slice and serve.

OPTIONS
• Bake the roast in an oven or convection oven at 325° to desired doneness.

Beef Roast with Burgundy Marinade

VERY LOW CARBOHYDRATES　　　　　　　　**NUMBER OF SERVINGS: 10 TO 12**

> *1 cup burgundy cooking wine*
> *½ cup olive oil*
> *2 tablespoons minced fresh parsley*
> *½ teaspoon dried tarragon*
> *½ teaspoon dried thyme*
> *1 bay leaf, crushed*
>
> *5-pound beef roast*

1. Combine the burgundy, olive oil, parsley, tarragon, thyme, and bay leaf.
2. Pour the marinade over the meat. Cover and refrigerate several hours or overnight, turning the roast several times.
3. Preheat oven or convection oven to 325°.
4. Remove the roast from the marinade and place on a rack in a roasting pan. Pour 1 or 2 cups of water in the bottom of the pan.
5. Bake uncovered to desired doneness. Add a little more water to the bottom, as needed.
6. Let sit on the counter for about 10 minutes, then slice and serve.

OPTIONS
- Drape two or three slices of bacon over the roast prior to baking.

3-Way Beef Roast: Grilled, Smoked or Baked

VERY LOW CARBOHYDRATES　　　　　　　　**NUMBER OF SERVINGS: 4**

> *1 tablespoon dry purchased barbecue spice blend*
> *¾ teaspoon paprika*
> *⅛ teaspoon black pepper*
> *2-pound beef roast*
>
> *½ cup Westbrae Unsweetened Un-Ketchup OR tomato sauce, if oven baking*
> *1 teaspoon hickory or pecan chips, if using the Cameron's Stovetop Smoker*

1. Combine the barbecue spice blend, paprika, and pepper. Rub all over the outside of the roast.

2. Wrap the roast in plastic, and refrigerate overnight or for 24 hours.
3. Remove the plastic and grill the roast outdoors on medium to low to desired doneness. Serve.

OPTIONS

- To smoke the roast, rub the barbecue spice blend, paprika and pepper over the meat, cut into 1-inch strips, and place in a single layer on the rack in the Cameron's Stovetop Smoker with 1 teaspoon of hickory or pecan chips. Turn the largest stovetop burner on medium heat and leave the lid cracked to ¼ inch. As soon as you see the first wisp of smoke, close the lid and begin timing. The meat is done in 20 minutes.
- To bake the roast, mix the barbecue spice blend, paprika, and pepper with ½ cup Westbrae Unsweetened Un-Ketchup or tomato sauce. Spread over the beef, and put ¼-inch of water in the pan. Cover, and bake in the oven at 350° for 1 to 2 hours or to desired doneness. When nearly done, cut the meat and immerse in the liquid in the roaster, cover, and return to the oven for another 30 minutes or so.

Beef Goulash

LOW CARBOHYDRATES   **NUMBER OF SERVINGS: 4 OR 5**

2 medium onions, chopped
¼ cup butter

2 pound rump roast cut into 2 inch cubes
  OR lean stew meat
1 clove garlic, minced
8-ounce can tomato sauce
1 teaspoon marjoram
¼ teaspoon salt

1. Cook the onion in the butter in a large, covered saucepan until transparent.
2. Add the meat and the remaining ingredients. Stir together. Cover and simmer on the stove for 2 hours; Uncover for the last 15 minutes if the sauce does not look thickened.
3. Serve garnished with a parsley sprig, if desired.

OPTIONS

- Add up to 1 tablespoon paprika OR chili powder.
- Add ¼ to ½ teaspoon caraway seeds.
- Simmer on low in the Crock-Pot all day.

> **I had a dish very similar to this in Germany and was surprised that their goulash had no pasta!**

Encore Beef Soup

LOW CARBOHYDRATES   **NUMBER OF SERVINGS: 4**

> **6 cups beef broth, homemade, canned or leftover beef juices from a roast, or a combination**
> **¾ cup diced onion**
> **Several diced mushrooms, if desired**
>
> **Salt and pepper to taste**
>
> **4 cups diced leftover beef roast or steak**
> **⅓ cup cooking sherry**

1. Heat the broth, onion, and mushrooms to a boil; cover and simmer until the onion is transparent.
2. Add the meat and cook for 5 minutes.
3. Add the sherry and serve.

> **Excellent and oh-so-quick—this soup can be made in 10 minutes!**
> **The Ulu Knife is wonderful for dicing or chopping, which is done with a rocking motion and is easy on the wrist.**

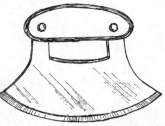

Basic Grilled Steak & Optional Homemade Steak Seasoning

NO CARBOHYDRATES   **NUMBER OF SERVINGS: AS DESIRED**

> **Beef steak (sirloin or another cut suitable for the grill)**
> **Olive oil (optional)**
> **Salt and pepper (optional)**
> **Herbs or herb blend, like Montreal Steak Blend, if desired (optional)**

1. Preheat the grill on high.
2. If the steak is ringed with fat, either remove it or slash through it every 2 inches to prevent shrinkage, which causes the meat to curl.
3. Coat the steak on all sides with olive oil. Sprinkle with salt and pepper or a favorite herb blend.

4. Place the steak on the grill, close the lid, and reduce the heat to medium or low, if using a less expensive steak cut.
5. Turn the meat once or twice.

OPTIONS
- Season the steak with Homemade Steak Seasoning:
  - 1 teaspoon paprika
  - 1 teaspoon garlic powder
  - 1 teaspoon onion powder
  - ½ teaspoon black pepper

Always turn the meat with tongs, never a fork, which will puncture the meat and allow the juices to run out.

In addition to the meat temperature test mentioned at the beginning of this section, some chefs use the touch test for steak:
- Rare meat gives easily when touched, but no juices appear on the surface.
- Medium meat feels firmer yet is somewhat springy, and some juices appear on the surface.
- Well-done meat is firm and covered with juices.
- Cook to desired doneness and serve.

Grilled Steak with Garlic Rub

VERY LOW CARBOHYDRATES   **NUMBER OF SERVINGS: 3**

1 pound sirloin steak OR Top of Iowa steak
3 or 4 cloves of garlic, minced
Softened butter, at room temperature

1. Rub the minced garlic onto all surfaces of the steak. Let sit a few minutes, or cover and refrigerate overnight.
2. Preheat grill on high.
3. Place the meat on the grill and reduce the heat. Brush steak top generously with the butter, top side only. Close the lid. When the bottom is browned, turn the steak and brush the top generously with butter. Cook to desired doneness and serve.

OPTIONS
- In place of the garlic and butter, substitute one of the butters listed for the Grilled Steak with Parsley Butter and 6 Variations (p. 68) and just brush it on as the steak is grilling.

My butcher tells me that Top of Iowa steak is the heart of the sirloin, trimmed and cut 1½ inches thick. It's wonderful.

Beef   **65**

Easy Grilled Steak with Worcestershire Butter Sauce

NO OR VERY LOW CARBOHYDRATES   NUMBER OF SERVINGS: 2

1 pound sirloin steak OR Top of Iowa steak OR other steak cut

1½ tablespoons butter, melted
¾ teaspoon Worcestershire sauce

1. Preheat the grill, broiler, or convection broiler on high.
2. Combine the butter and Worcestershire sauce and brush on all sides of the steak.
3. Place the meat on the grill and close the lid. Reduce the heat to medium or medium low and cook the steak to desired doneness, turning occasionally, and serve.

> Some people think you should only turn a steak once; perhaps this is true for rare steaks. But we prefer ours medium and well-done, and Bob feels that the juices stay in better if they're turned several times.

Grilled Steak with 2 Melted Butter Sauces

VERY LOW CARBOHYDRATES   NUMBER OF SERVINGS: 3

1½ pound Top of Iowa steak OR other steak
Olive oil

Barbecue Butter Sauce (see below)

1. Preheat the grill on high.
2. Generously coat the steak with olive oil. Place on the grill, close the lid and reduce the heat to medium. Cook to desired doneness, turning the meat once or twice.

Barbecue Butter Sauce:

¼ cup butter
1½ teaspoon Westbrae Unsweetened Un-Ketchup
1½ teaspoons no carb Worcestershire sauce
2 green onions, chopped, including tops
⅛ teaspoon salt

Back to Protein

3. Place all of the ingredients in a small cast-iron skillet (6 inches in diameter.) Put the skillet on the grill when steaks are nearly done to melt the butter and heat through sauce OR melt the butter and heat the sauce in a Pyrex measuring cup in the microwave.

4. Prepare the butter sauce, then pour over the cooked meat and serve.

OPTIONS

• An alternate butter sauce recipe is Garlic Butter Sauce:
> ¼ cup butter
> 1 or 2 cloves minced garlic
> ⅛ teaspoon salt

Grilled Steak with Parsley Butter + 6 Variations

TRACE CARBOHYDRATES   **NUMBER OF SERVINGS: 2 OR 3**

1 to 1½ pounds Top of Iowa steak
Olive oil (optional)

Parsley Butter (recipe below)

1. Heat the grill on high.
2. Rub the steak with the olive oil (optional).
3. Place the strip of meat on the grill, close the lid, and turn the heat down to medium. After about 7 minutes, turn the meat and salt and pepper the browned side. Repeat. Cook to desired doneness.
4. Serve the steak with mounds of parsley butter on top. Wonderful!

Parsley Butter Sauce:

> *3 tablespoons butter, softened*
> *3 tablespoons minced fresh parsley*
> *Salt and pepper to taste*

5. Wash the parsley and cut the heads off of the stems. Mince the parsley on a cutting board with a rotary mincer. Put the butter in a coffee cup, add the parsley. Blend with a fork. If desired, form into a shape and chill; otherwise, use immediately.

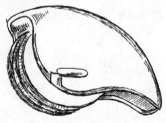

OPTIONS

Here are some more butter recipes:

• Chives Butter
> 4 tablespoons softened butter
> 2 tablespoons finely chopped chives

- Garlic Butter
    - 4 tablespoons softened butter
    - 1 clove minced garlic
    - ½ teaspoon minced fresh parsley
    - ¼ teaspoon salt

- Herb Butter
    - 4 tablespoons softened butter
    - ½ tablespoon fresh minced basil, marjoram, rosemary, thyme OR ½ teaspoon dried basil, chili powder, garlic powder, paprika, savory, marjoram, mustard, rosemary, or thyme

- Lemon Parsley Butter
    - 4 tablespoons softened butter
    - 2 teaspoons lemon juice
    - 1 tablespoon minced fresh parsley
    - dash salt and pepper

- Paprika Butter
    - 4 tablespoons softened butter
    - ½ teaspoon paprika
    - ¼ teaspoon onion salt
    - 1 clove garlic, minced

- Tarragon Butter
    - 4 tablespoons softened butter
    - 1 tablespoon minced fresh parsley
    - 1 tablespoon finely chopped chives
    - 1 tablespoon minced shallots or onion
    - 1 teaspoon dried tarragon

Grilled Steak with Whipped Cream

VERY LOW CARBOHYDRATES   **NUMBER OF SERVINGS: 3**

3 slices thick bacon
1½ pounds sirloin steak OR Top of Iowa steak

½ cup heavy cream
1 or 2 green onions, diced OR 2 table-
    spoons chives, diced
1 red radish, diced fine plus additional thin
    slices for garnish

1. Cook the bacon in a skillet. When very crisp, drain on paper towels.
2. Preheat a grill or broiler on high. Cook the steaks to desired doneness, turning occasionally.

3. Whip the cream until very stiff. (The Cuisinart Hand Blender is great for this job.) Fold in the green onions and the radish.
4. Serve the steak with a generous dollop of the whipped cream mixture, crumble and sprinkle the bacon over all. Garnish with radish slices, if desired.

> Radishes and onions grow quickly, and can take a little frost, so they can be planted very early in the spring. And they're wonderful in this recipe!

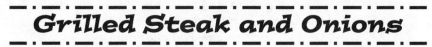

Grilled Steak and Onions

LOW CARBOHYDRATES   **NUMBER OF SERVINGS: 2**

Olive oil
2 large onions, sliced thickly
1 pound sirloin steak OR Top of Iowa steak

1. Preheat the grill on high.
2. Generously grease a large cast-iron skillet with the olive oil. If your skillet has a wooden handle, remove the wood part by unscrewing the end. Dump the onion slices in the skillet, and place the skillet on the hot grill. Close the lid.
3. After 5 or 6 minutes, turn the heat down to medium, add the steak on the grill, and close the lid. Stir the onions occasionally; turn the meat once or twice. Cook the meat to desired doneness and the onions until they're well-browned.
4. Serve the steak topped with onions. Wonderful!

OPTIONS
• Use only 1 onion and add 8 ounces of sliced mushrooms to the onions in the skillet.

> • A well-seasoned, cast iron skillet is a treasure; care for it well. Never put a cast-iron skillet in the dishwasher. Always wash by hand with very little detergent and dry thoroughly or the skillet will rust.
> • Hand wash your cast-iron cookware, pat it dry; rub the inside with olive oil, then place on a burner on low heat to be sure it's thoroughly dry and seasoned.

Grilled Steak and Cheese

VERY LOW CARBOHYDRATES   **NUMBER OF SERVINGS: 2**

> 1 pound Top of Iowa beef steak OR beef
>   tenderloin
> Salt and pepper
>
> 1 tablespoon finely grated Parmesan
>   cheese
> 3 tablespoons finely shredded soft cheese,
>   such as smoked cheddar
> 1 garlic clove OR ¼ teaspoon garlic herb
>   blend, like garlic with parsley (both
>   optional)
>
> 2 or 3 tablespoons chopped green onion,
>   including tops OR 1 or 2 tablespoons
>   chopped chives

1. Preheat the grill on high.
2. Sprinkle salt and pepper on each side of the steak. Place the steak on the grill, close the lid, and reduce the heat to medium. Grill to desired doneness.
3. Preheat the broiler on high.
4. Combine the Parmesan, cheddar, and garlic. Place the cheeses on top of the steak. Put the steak under the broiler for a minute or so until the cheeses melt and started to brown—be sure to watch it carefully.
5. Remove the steak from the broiler, top with the chopped onions or chives, and serve.

> This is our all-time favorite grilled steak recipe! Absolutely wonderful!

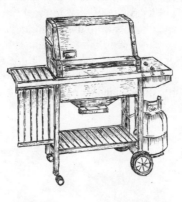

Grilled Steak with Horseradish Cream

VERY LOW CARBOHYDRATES   **NUMBER OF SERVINGS: 3**

> 1½ pounds sirloin steak OR Top of Iowa
> steak
>
> ½ cup heavy cream
> 2 to 3 tablespoons horseradish
> Salt (optional)
>
> Parsley for garnish (optional)

1. Preheat the grill or broiler on high.
2. Cook steaks to desired doneness, turning occasionally.
3. Whip the cream until very stiff. (The Cuisinart Hand Blender is great for this job.) Fold in the horseradish and salt, if desired.
4. Serve the steak with a generous dollop of horseradish cream. Garnish with a sprig of parsley.

> Even people who don't like horseradish will love this! The idea for the recipe came from a cookbook dating near the turn of the century—1900, not 2000!

Grilled Filet Mignon

NO CARBOHYDRATES   **NUMBER OF SERVINGS: 2**

> Beef tenderloin for two (about 1 pound),
> sliced 1- to 1¼-inches thick (or cut your
> own from a whole tenderloin)
> 2 thick slices of bacon (check the label for
> no added sugar)
> Salt and pepper, if desired

1. Heat the grill on high.
2. Trim only excess fat from the tenderloins.
3. For each serving, wrap a piece of bacon around the fillet and secure with a toothpick.
4. Grill on low to medium heat, to desired doneness, and serve.

OPTIONS
- Hickory-smoked bacon is wonderful in this recipe. To smoke your own, see page 95.

Easy Grilled Sirloin with Marinade

NO CARBOHYDRATES   **NUMBER OF SERVINGS: 2**

> ¼ *cup no-carb soy sauce*
> ¼ *cup no-carb Worcestershire sauce*
> *1 pound sirloin steak OR Top of Iowa steak*

1. Combine the soy sauce and the Worcestershire sauce and pour over the steak, coating it on all sides. Marinate in the refrigerator for 2 to 3 hours.
2. Preheat grill (or broiler) on high. Put the steaks on, close the lid, and turn the heat down to medium and cook to desired doneness, turning occasionally.

OPTIONS
- Serve with a sprinkle of garlic powder or a coarse ground garlic/parsley blend seasoning.

Grilled Steak Marinated in Beer

LOW CARBOHYDRATES   **NUMBER OF SERVINGS: 2 OR 3**

> *12-ounce can Miller Lite Beer*
> *3 tablespoons dried onion flakes*
> ½ *teaspoon cumin*
> *2 cloves garlic, minced OR* ¼ *teaspoon garlic powder*
>
> *1-pound steak*

1. Combine the beer, onion, cumin, and garlic. Pour the marinade over the steak, cover, and refrigerate for 12 hours.
2. Preheat the grill or broiler on high. Put the steaks on and turn the heat down to medium. Discard the marinade. Cook to desired doneness, turning occasionally.

Grilled Steak with Horseradish & Worcestershire Marinade

NUMBER OF SERVINGS: 2

> **2 tablespoons soy sauce**
> **1 tablespoon Worcestershire sauce**
> **1½ teaspoons horseradish**
> **1 clove garlic, minced OR 1 teaspoon garlic powder**
>
> **1 pound sirloin tip OR steak of choice**

1. Combine the soy sauce, Worcestershire sauce, horseradish, and garlic in a coffeecup.
2. Coat the steak on all sides, pour the remaining sauce on top. Cover and refrigerate for 2 hours or so.
3. Preheat grill on high.
4. Place the steak on the grill, close the lid, and reduce the heat to medium. Turn once or twice and baste with marinade. Cook to desired doneness and serve.

Tangy Marinated Steak on the Grill

NUMBER OF SERVINGS: 3

> **¼ cup olive oil**
> **1 tablespoon fresh parsley, finely minced**
> **1½ tablespoons lemon juice**
> **1 tablespoon vinegar**
> **1 tablespoon no-carb soy sauce**
> **1 tablespoon no-carb Worcestershire sauce**
> **1 teaspoon dry mustard**
> **½ teaspoon black pepper**
> **½ teaspoon salt**
> **1 clove garlic, minced**
>
> **1½ pounds sirloin steak OR Top of Iowa steak**

1. Combine all of the ingredients except the steak. Blend well in a food processor or blender.

2. Pour the marinade over the meat. Cover and refrigerate overnight or prepare in the morning before work and marinate all day to grill for supper.
3. Preheat the grill on high. Remove the meat from the marinade and
place on the grill. Close the lid and reduce the heat to medium. Cook
to desired doneness and serve.

Steak Tamer Marinade for the Grill

VERY LOW CARBOHYDRATES   **NUMBER OF SERVINGS: 2**

⅓ cup olive oil
2 tablespoons red wine vinegar
2 teaspoons dried onion flakes
1 teaspoon celery salt
1 teaspoon prepared horseradish
½ teaspoon dry mustard
½ teaspoon black pepper
Dash garlic powder

1 pound round steak or other cheaper cut

1. Combine all of the ingredients and mix well. Pour the marinade over
the meat, cover, and refrigerate overnight or all day.
2. Preheat the grill on high.
3. Remove the meat from the marinade and place on the grill. Close the
lid and reduce the heat to medium. Turn meat occasionally, brushing
on more marinade until the meat is nearly done. Cook to desired
doneness and serve.

Grilled Steak with Rosemary Marinade

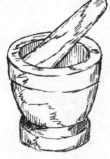

VERY LOW CARBOHYDRATES   **NUMBER OF SERVINGS: 2**

2 tablespoons olive oil
2 tablespoons soy sauce
2 tablespoons red cooking wine
2 or 3 large garlic cloves, minced
½ teaspoon rosemary, crushed
Dash of black pepper and salt

1 pound beef steak of choice

1. Combine all of the ingredients except the steak; pour over the meat. Cover and refrigerate overnight or from 4 to 12 hours.
2. Preheat the grill on high.
3. Remove the steak from the marinade and place on the grill. Close the lid and turn the heat down to medium. Turn the meat once or twice. Cook to desired doneness and serve.

> To crush rosemary, place the dried herb in a mortar and pestle and grind with a circular motion. In this recipe, adding the salt to the rosemary aides the crushing action.

Grilled Steak with Mustard Marinade

VERY LOW CARBOHYDRATES   **NUMBER OF SERVINGS: 2**

1 pound steak of choice
1 tablespoon Dijon mustard OR prepared mustard

2 tablespoons burgundy cooking wine
2 tablespoons lemon juice
2 tablespoons soy sauce
2 tablespoons Worcestershire sauce

1. Rub the mustard into both sides of the steak.
2. Combine the wine, lemon juice, soy sauce, and Worcestershire sauce. Pour over the meat, coating all sides. Cover and refrigerate for 4 to 12 hours.
3. Preheat the grill on high.
4. Remove the meat from the marinade and place on the grill. Close the lid and reduce the heat to medium. Turn once or twice. Cook to desired doneness and serve.

Grilled Whiskey Kabobs

¼ cup whiskey
¼ cup soy sauce
2 tablespoons olive oil
2 teaspoons lemon juice
1 clove garlic, minced
¼ teaspoon black pepper

1½ pounds beef steak, trimmed of excess fat
    and cut into 1½-inch chunks

1 green pepper, cut into 1 inch chunks
6 fresh mushrooms
1 onion, cut into 1 inch chunks

1. Combine the whiskey, soy sauce, olive oil, lemon juice, garlic and black pepper and pour over the steak chunks. Cover and refrigerate for 4 to 8 hours.
2. Preheat the grill on high.
3. Assemble skewers, alternating steak chunks and vegetable. Brush the kabobs with the remaining marinade.
4. Coat a grill rack with vegetable oil spray. Place the skewers on the grill, close the lid, and reduce the heat to medium. Turn the skewers often, basting after 10 minutes with additional marinade. Cook until the meat is at a desired doneness and serve.

Do NOT refrigerate the vegetables with the meat in the marinade; the mushrooms will soak up the liquid and turn mushy.

For wooden skewers, soak in water 30 minutes prior to grilling to prevent charring OR use metal skewers. If the skewers have wooden handles, be sure to position the skewers so that the handles are off the hot grill.

Encore Steak and Sour Cream

LOW CARBOHYDRATES   **NUMBER OF SERVINGS: VARIABLE**

Sliced mushrooms and/or sliced onions
Butter
Leftover steak
Sour cream

1. In a small skillet, saute a few sliced mushrooms and onion slices in a little butter.
2. Slice the leftover steak into thin strips, sprinkle with a little water, and microwave until hot.
3. Serve the steak covered with the mushrooms and onions. Top everything with a dollop of sour cream.

OPTIONS
- Serve on a bed of lettuce, as a hot salad.

These recipes are quick and easy!

Encore Grilled Steak with Burgundy Cream

VERY LOW CARBOHYDRATES   **NUMBER OF SERVINGS: 2**

1 tablespoon melted butter
About 1 pound leftover grilled steak, cut
into bite-sized strips
¼ cup diced onion

2 to 3 tablespoons burgundy cooking wine
2 tablespoons heavy whipping cream
Salt and pepper as desired

1. Melt the butter in a skillet. Add the steak and onions. Cook together until the onion is transparent and the meat is heated through.
2. Add the burgundy and simmer for 2 minutes.
3. Add the cream and let bubble as it simmers without stirring for 2 minutes.
4. Salt and pepper to taste and serve.

OPTIONS
- Add a few mushrooms with the onions.
- Use leftover roast meat instead of the steak.

Beef   **77**

Encore Italian Steak Salad

LOW CARBOHYDRATES   **NUMBER OF SERVINGS: VARIABLE**

> Lettuce, torn up
> Leftover steak, thinly sliced and cut into
>   bite-sized pieces
>
> Diced onion OR green onion, including tops,
>   2 tablespoons per serving
> Dash garlic powder
> 2 or 3 black olives, sliced, per serving
> Olive oil and red wine vinegar (about twice
>   as much olive oil as the vinegar)
> Grated Parmesan cheese; one or two table-
>   spoons per serving

Assemble ingredients in salad bowls in the order given, and serve.

OPTIONS
- Add sweet red or green peppers or sliced pepperoni to the salad.
- The meat can be served hot or cold.

Smoked Steak

VERY LOW CARBOHYDRATES   **NUMBER OF SERVINGS: 2 OR 3**

> 1 teaspoon cherry wood chips OR chips of choice
> 1 pound Top of Iowa steaks OR beef cut of
>   choice, cut into long strips about 1 inch
>   by 1 inch
> Red cooking wine (optional)
> Steak herb blend of choice OR Homemade
>   Steak Seasoning, see "Basic Grilled
>   Steak," p. 65

1. Place the wood chips in the bottom of a Camerons Stovetop Smoker. Place the drip tray and rack over the chips. Lay the steak strips on the rack. Drizzle the wine over the meat; sprinkle with the herbs, if desired.
2. Slide on the lid, leaving it barely cracked open. Place the Smoker on the largest burner on your stove; turn the heat to medium.
3. As soon as you see the first wisp of smoke escape from the Smoker, close the lid and begin the timing. Cooking takes 20 minutes; do not overcook.

OPTIONS
- This amount of wood chips works well for up to 2 pounds of steak.

Back to Protein

Oak Smoked Beef Tenderloin

NO CARBOHYDRATES   **NUMBER OF SERVINGS: 2**

1 tablespoon olive oil
½ teaspoon basil
Dash salt and pepper

1 pound beef tenderloin, cut into 4 slices

1 tablespoon Camerons oak chips

1. Combine the olive oil, basil, salt, and pepper and rub on the meat.
2. Place the wood chips in the bottom of a Camerons Stovetop Smoker. Place the drip tray and rack over the chips. Lay the meat on the rack. Slide on the lid, leaving it barely cracked open. Place the Smoker on the largest burner on your stove; turn the heat to medium.
3. As soon as you see the first wisp of smoke escape from the Smoker, close the lid and begin the timing. Cooking takes 20 minutes; do not overcook.

Basic Stovetop Steak

NO CARBOHYDRATES   **NUMBER OF SERVINGS: 2**

1 to 2 tablespoons butter
1 pound beef tenderloin OR steak of choice
Salt and pepper as desired

⅓ cup water OR broth OR wine

1. Melt the butter in a skillet, add the steak, and saute on medium heat till until both sides are browned and the meat is done.
2. Add the water, broth, or wine and simmer on the lowest setting. Scrape up the browned bits on the bottom of the skillet; this takes only a minute or two while the liquid is reduced.
3. Serve the meat with any remaining liquid on top.

OPTIONS

- Add a few sliced mushrooms to the skillet before adding the liquid.
- Add a few onion slices to the skillet before adding the liquid.
- Add ¼ teaspoon dried herb or herb combination of your choice to the liquid.

Brandy Steak and Shallots

1 to 2 tablespoons butter
1 shallot clove, cut into slivers
1 pound steak (I use Top of Iowa cut in
strips, but it could be a fillet left whole
or any cheaper steak cut into bite-sized
pieces)
Salt and pepper as desired
2 tablespoons brandy or red cooking wine
(only a small trace of carb)

1. Melt the butter in a medium skillet on medium heat and add the shallot slivers. Stir-fry together about one minute. Push to one side of the pan.
2. Add the steak, salt, and pepper and cook about 2 minutes. Then turn over and continue cooking to a desired doneness. Remove the meat to a serving platter.
3. Add the brandy to the skillet, stirring quickly for about 30 seconds. Pour brandy-shallots over the steak and serve.

OPTIONS
* Rub minced garlic or herbs of choice into the steak.

This is so easy and delicious!

Southwest Beef

1 pound sirloin steak, sliced thin, OR anoth-
er steak cut
¾ teaspoon purchased fajita spice blend OR
purchased mesquite seasoning
Juice from 1 lime and reserve zest

1 tablespoon olive oil
1 medium green bell pepper, cut into bite-
sized chunks
½ medium red sweet pepper, cut into bite-
sized chunks

½ medium onion, cut into bite-sized chunks

Sour cream

Reserved lime zest

1. Remove the zest from the lime; reserve for later.
2. Combine the steak, spice blend, and lime juice. Marinate for 1 hour.
3. Heat olive oil in a wok or skillet on high heat. Add the steak strips and any remaining lime juice. Stir fry 1 or 2 minutes, then add the peppers and onions. Stir-fry until steak is done and the vegetables are tender-crisp.
4. Serve with a dollop of sour cream and sprinkle zest of lime over all.

Steak Stir Fry with Green Peppers, Bean Sprouts, and Tomato

LOW CARBOHYDRATES   **NUMBER OF SERVINGS: 2 OR 3**

1 tablespoon peanut OR olive oil
1 pound steak, trimmed of excess fat and sliced into ¼-inch by 1½-inch strips
1 clove garlic, minced
Gingerroot, 1 inch in diameter by ¼ inch, finely chopped
Dash pepper

1 tablespoon soy sauce
1 medium green pepper, chopped into bite-sized pieces
1 cup bean sprouts

1 medium tomato, skinned, seeded, and cut into 1-inch pieces

1. Place the oil in a wok on high heat. Add the meat strips, garlic, gingerroot, and pepper and stir-fry for about 5 minutes, or until the meat is browned.
2. Add the soy sauce, green pepper and bean sprouts; and stir-fry for 2 to 3 minutes.
3. Add the tomato and stir-fry another minute or two, then serve.

> • To make slicing the steak into strips easier, partially freeze the meat first.
> • Peanut oil takes high heat without smoking.

Beef "Sukiyaki"

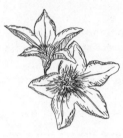

1 tablespoon oil

1 pound beef steak, trimmed of excess fat and cut into 1 inch strips

¾ cup chopped onion OR 6 green onions, chopped, including tops

2 ribs celery, sliced thin and at an angle

4 ounces sliced fresh mushrooms

4 ounces canned water chestnuts, drained and sliced in half

¼ cup double strength beef bouillon OR water plus ½ teaspoon instant beef granules

¼ cup soy sauce

2 tablespoons vermouth

1 to 1½ cups packed fresh spinach that has been chopped into ½ inch strips

1. Heat the oil in a skillet and brown the steak strips, stirring constantly.
2. Add the onion, celery, mushrooms, and water chestnuts. Stir-fry about 5 minutes.
3. Pour in the broth, soy sauce, and vermouth. Simmer 5 minutes. Most of the liquid will be gone.
4. Toss in the spinach and stir-fry about 2 minutes, or just until the spinach wilts. Serve in a pretty bowl.

OPTIONS

- Increase the amount of spinach to 2 cups, if desired.
- Garnish each serving with a squash blossom picked fresh from your garden and sauteed a short while in a little butter. Attractive and delicious!

When entertaining, I like to serve this dish along with "Asparagus Chicken" (see p. 170). for contrasting yet complimentary main dishes. Have the ingredients prepared ahead of time and cook in front of the guests, or let them stir—it takes very little time and makes a low-stress meal.

Easy Stovetop Italian Round Steak

VERY LOW CARBOHYDRATES   **NUMBER OF SERVINGS: 4**

¾ **cup tomato sauce**
1½ **teaspoons thyme**
2 **cloves garlic, minced**
½ **teaspoon salt, if desired**

1½ **pounds round steak OR other cheaper
    cut, cut into 2-inch squares**
1 **to 2 tablespoons butter OR olive oil**

1. Cook the tomato sauce, thyme, garlic and salt together on the stove for 5 minutes OR heat in the microwave, covered, for 2 minutes.
2. Brown the steak on both sides in a skillet in the melted butter. Pour the sauce over the meat. Cover and cook slowly at a simmer until the steak is tender. Serve.

This came from Aunt Nell's cookbook, dated about 1900.

Baked Italian Steak

LOW CARBOHYDRATES   **NUMBER OF SERVINGS: 4 OR 5**

1½ **to 2 pound sirloin steak**

½ **cup water**
14-**ounce can tomatoes in juice (check the
    label for no added sugar) OR 2 or 3
    fresh tomatoes, peeled and seeded and
    cut into bite-sized chunks**
1 **teaspoon oregano**
2 **cloves garlic, minced**

1. Preheat the oven to 350°.
2. Place the water and the steak in a large oven-proof skillet. Add the tomatoes, oregano, and garlic. Stir together on top of the meat.
3. Cover with a tight-fitting lid or seal with aluminum foil. Bake for 30 to 40 minutes, then uncover and bake another 10 minutes, or until the meat is brown but not dry.

OPTIONS
- Although unnecessary, you can brown the sirloin steak in 2 tablespoons of butter before adding the other ingredients.

Beef   83

Oriental Pepper Steak

LOW CARBOHYDRATES   **NUMBER OF SERVINGS: 4 TO 5**

> *1½ pound beef steak of choice, cut into thin*
> *strips*
> *3 tablespoons olive oil*
> *1 cup beef broth (canned or homemade)*
> *¼ teaspoon minced gingerroot*
> *1 teaspoon soy sauce*
> *2 tomatoes, peeled and cut into wedges*
> *1 green sweet pepper, cut into strips*
> *1 medium onion, cut into bite-sized chunks*
> *4 or 5 sliced mushrooms (optional)*

1. Put the olive oil in a skillet on high heat. Add the beef and brown, stir-ring constantly.
2. Add the broth, gingerroot, and soy sauce. Bring to a boil, then reduce the heat and simmer 15 minutes, uncovered.
3. Add the tomatoes, green pepper, onion, and mushrooms. Stir together and simmer until the liquid is reduced, vegetables are crisp-tender, and the meat is tender. Serve with the remaining liquid.

OPTIONS

• For "American Pepper Steak," omit the gingerroot and soy sauce.

Steak Baked with Lemon & Onions

LOW CARBOHYDRATES   **NUMBER OF SERVINGS: 3**

> *1½ pound Top of Iowa OR sirloin steak*
> *Salt and pepper*
> *½ teaspoon dry mustard*
> *½ teaspoon Worcestershire sauce*
>
> *2 tablespoons Westbrae Unsweetened Un-*
> *Ketchup*
> *Hungarian paprika OR paprika*
> *1 onion, sliced*
> *1 lemon, sliced*
>
> *3 tablespoons butter*

1. Sprinkle salt and pepper onto both sides of the steak. Mix together the dry mustard and Worcestershire sauce into a paste; rub into

both sides of the steak. Cut the steak into thick strips, 1 inch by 1½ inch. Place in a baking dish.

2. Preheat the oven to 375° Or a convection oven to 350°.
3. Brush the top of the meat with Un-Ketchup. Sprinkle with paprika. Place the onion slices on top of the steak and top with the lemon slices. (Discard the end slices from the lemon; it has too much white pith and will turn bitter.)
4. Bake, uncovered, for about 75 minutes or to desired doneness OR convection oven bake about 1 hour to desired doneness. Remove lemon slices, dot with butter, and serve.

OPTIONS
• You can assemble this dish and refrigerate overnight or all day until needed, say for supper after a work day.

Beef in Beer Sauce

LOW CARBOHYDRATES   **NUMBER OF SERVINGS: 2**

> 1 pound beef steak of choice, trimmed of
>   excess fat
> 1 to 2 tablespoons butter or oil
>
> 1 medium onion
> 1 clove garlic, minced
>
> ¾ cup beef broth
> ¾ cup Miller Lite Beer
> 4 ounce can sliced mushrooms plus liquid
> 3 tablespoons Westbrae Unsweetened Un-
>   Ketchup
> 1 bay leaf
> ¼ teaspoon pepper

1. Melt the butter in a skillet, and lightly brown the steak on both sides on medium heat.
2. Add the onion and garlic and brown with the steak, stirring often.
3. Add the broth, beer, mushrooms, Un-Ketchup, bay leaf, and pepper. Cover and simmer 1 hour or more; remove the lid for the last 20 minutes to reduce the liquid.
4. Remove the bay leaf and serve the steak with the sauce.

OPTIONS
• Cubed stew meat can be substituted for the steak. After the meat and onions are browned, put all ingredients in a Crock-Pot for half a day on high or all day on low——the latter is better.

A cheaper cut of steak can be used for this recipe.

Stovetop Round Steak and Onions

LOW CARBOHYDRATES   **NUMBER OF SERVINGS: 3**

2 or 3 tablespoons butter
2 medium onions, sliced

1½ pound round steak, OR other steak, cut into
    strips 2 or 3 inches long and ½ inch wide

1 cup beef broth OR water
1 tablespoon vinegar OR lemon juice
2 cloves garlic, minced (optional)
1 bay leaf (optional)
¼ teaspoon thyme (optional)
Salt and pepper as desired

1. Melt the butter in a large skillet, add the onions, and cook on medium heat until browned.
2. Add the steak strips to the skillet and cook until the steak is browned.
3. Add the remaining ingredients and bring to a boil. Reduce the heat and cover; simmer 45 minute to 1 hour.
4. Most of the liquid will be evaporated, but what is left will be like a gravy—serve it with the meat and onions.

OPTIONS

• Eliminate the lemon juice or vinegar and pour ⅓ cup red cooking wine plus ⅓ cup olive oil over the steak strips; refrigerate for several hours, if possible. This will tenderize the meat.

Top of Iowa Steak and Onions on the Stove

LOW CARBOHYDRATES   **NUMBER OF SERVINGS: 3**

1½ pounds sirloin tip steak, OR Top of Iowa
Salt and pepper
¼ cup butter
1 medium onion, sliced
¾ cup red cooking wine

1. Rub salt and pepper into the steak.
2. Melt the butter in a skillet. Add the meat and brown on both sides.

Reduce the heat to a simmer. Place onion slices over meat; pour wine over all. Cover tightly and simmer on lowest heat for 2 hours or to desired doneness.

3. Serve with onions and remaining liquid.

Easy Boneless Round Steak and Sauce

VERY LOW CARBOHYDRATES   **NUMBER OF SERVINGS: 2**

> **1 pound boneless round steak OR other cheaper cut**
> **Dash salt and pepper**
> **2 tablespoons butter**
> **¾ cup beef broth, homemade OR canned**
> **½ cup heavy cream**
> **1 tablespoon Worcestershire sauce OR Westbrae Unsweetened Un-Ketchup (optional)**

1. Trim the steak of excess fat; cut into serving-size pieces. Sprinkle a little salt and pepper on both sides.
2. Melt the butter in a skillet. Add the steak pieces and cook on low, turning occasionally, until all liquids are absorbed and the meat is browned.
3. Add the beef broth and simmer on low, covered, for 45 minutes to an hour. This makes the cheaper cut of beef tender.
4. Remove the lid and reduce the liquid to half the original amount, (if not reduced already).
5. Add the cream and Worcestershire sauce or Un-Ketchup; simmer about 5 minutes until thickened.
6. Serve steak the topped with sauce.

OPTIONS

• If you choose not to use the Worcestershire sauce or Un-Ketchup, use double-strength canned broth for added flavor.

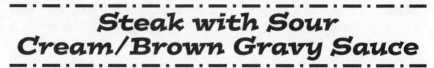

Steak with Sour Cream/Brown Gravy Sauce

VERY LOW CARBOHYDRATES   **NUMBER OF SERVINGS: 3 OR 4**

1½ pound beef steak, Top of Iowa, OR
  Tenderloin Fillet
2 tablespoons butter

2 tablespoons brandy
½ cup sour cream
2 tablespoons Westbrae Unsweetened Un-
  Ketchup
¼ teaspoons Worcestershire sauce
2 drops Tabasco sauce (we use the mild)
Dash of dried thyme

1. Melt the butter in a skillet and cook the steak to desired doneness, turning to brown both sides.
2. Remove the steak and keep warm.
3. Deglaze the skillet—pour in the brandy and stir to loosen the browned bits. Add the sour cream, Un-Ketchup, Worcestershire sauce, Tabasco sauce, and thyme; stir well. Return the steak to the skillet and heat through.
4. Serve the steak with sauce.

Easy Beef Tenderloin Steak and Sauce—Quick!

VERY LOW CARBOHYDRATES   **NUMBER OF SERVINGS: 2**

1 pound beef tenderloin fillet
Dash salt and pepper
1 to 2 tablespoons butter

½ cup beef broth, homemade OR canned
½ cup heavy cream
1 tablespoon Worcestershire sauce OR
  Westbrae Unsweetened Un-Ketchup
  (optional)

1. Sprinkle a little salt and pepper on both sides of the steak.
2. Melt the butter in a skillet. Add the fillet and cook on medium-low, until the meat is browned on both sides, about 3 minutes.
3. Add the beef broth and simmer on low, uncovered, about 10 minutes,

turning the meat once. The liquid should be reduced by half; if not, cook a little longer until it is.

4. Add the cream and Worcestershire sauce and simmer until thickened, about 5 minutes.
5. Serve the steak topped with the sauce.

OPTIONS

• Instead of the Worcestershire sauce or Un-Ketchup, use double-strength canned broth for added flavor.

• Wrap a slice of bacon around the outside of a fillet, fasten with a short metal skewer or toothpick that has been soaked in water, then grill to desired doneness for another taste delight!

> Beef tenderloin fillets are cheaper if you buy the whole tenderloin, with the strap, from your butcher. Trim off and discard the grisly strap; slice the meat crosswise into 6-to 8-ounce fillets. If you don't want to cook all of them at once, freeze some for later use.

Tenderloin with Caper Cream Sauce

LOW CARBOHYDRATES   **NUMBER OF SERVINGS: 2**

1 pound beef tenderloin, cut into 4 fillets
1½ tablespoons lemon juice
¼ teaspoon paprika
Dash black pepper

2 tablespoons butter
1½ tablespoons capers, drained

¼ cup white cooking wine
1 bay leaf
½ cup heavy cream

1. Dribble the lemon juice over the beef. Sprinkle with the paprika and pepper.
2. Melt the butter in a medium skillet. Add the fillets and the capers and cook on medium heat, cooking to desired doneness. Remove fillets to a small skillet on lowest heat to keep warm.
3. Add the wine and the bay leaf to the skillet with the capers. Simmer on medium heat for 2 or 3 minutes, scraping bottom of skillet to loosen browned bits.
4. Add the heavy cream and bring to a simmer, cooking on low till thickened without stirring. Remove bay leaf.
5. Serve the steaks with caper cream sauce spooned over meat.

OPTIONS

• Instead of capers, you can use 2 or 3 chopped green onions, including the tops.

Beef   **89**

Mock Beef Stroganoff

2 tablespoons butter
1 large onion, sliced thin
8 ounces mushrooms, sliced

2 tablespoons additional butter
1½ pounds beef tenderloin OR Top of Iowa
    steak, cut into strips about ½ inch thick

¾ cup sour cream
Freshly grated nutmeg, to taste (optional)
Salt and pepper, as desired (optional)

1. Melt 2 tablespoons butter in a skillet on high. Add the onion and mushrooms and reduce heat to medium high. Stir constantly until the onions are transparent and partially browned.
2. Add 2 tablespoons additional butter to the skillet. Toss in the meat strips and stir-fry on medium high for 5 minutes, or until the meat is browned on all sides; stir constantly.
3. Add the sour cream, nutmeg, salt, and pepper. Stir well, heat through, and serve.

For a cheaper version of this dish, see the "Mock Beef Stroganoff Stew," p. 53.

Steak Diane

1 tablespoon olive oil
1 or 2 cloves garlic, minced
1 tablespoon shallot, minced OR onion

2 beef tenderloin fillets
1 or 2 tablespoons Dijon mustard
black pepper

3 tablespoons butter
Several mushrooms, sliced

¼ cup burgundy
⅓ cup canned or homemade beef broth
Dash thyme
Pinch dried parsley

⅓ cup heavy cream

Back to Protein

1. Heat the olive oil in a skillet. Add the garlic and shallot or onion; cook until browned.
2. Add the fillets to the skillet and slather with mustard. When blood comes to the surface of the meat, turn, and sprinkle the top with freshly ground black pepper. Cook until the meat is nearly to desired doneness (check by slicing halfway into the meat and looking inside.)
3. Add the butter to the skillet. When the butter is melted, add the sliced mushrooms. Stir occasionally; cook until the mushrooms are done.
4. Add the burgundy, beef broth, thyme and parsley, and cook till reduced by half.
5. Add the cream and bring to a low boil, without stirring. Let simmer until the cream thickens, then stir to mix all the ingredients.
6. Serve the steak topped with the sauce and mushrooms. Fantastic!

My husband arranged to have Steak Diane at a special restaurant one romantic Valentine's Day. Later on, I was able to take gourmet cooking classes from the chef who shared his recipe, from which I've adapted this. Add a fresh salad, and you have a wonderful meal!

Mock Beef Wellington

LOW CARBOHYDRATES   **NUMBER OF SERVINGS: 2**

2, 6- to 8-ounce beef tenderloin fillets
1 clove garlic, minced
1 tablespoon butter

1 tablespoon additional butter
¼ cup finely minced shallots OR onion, minced
4 ounces sliced fresh mushrooms
2 tablespoons minced fresh parsley OR 2 teaspoons dried minced parsley

2 teaspoons Dijon mustard
⅛ teaspoon thyme
⅛ teaspoon salt
⅛ teaspoon pepper
½ cup beef broth (canned or homemade)
3 tablespoons burgundy cooking wine

2 eggs, separated
2 tablespoons finely grated American cheese OR cheese of choice

1. Preheat oven to 350°.
2. Rub the garlic into the meat.
3. Melt the butter in a small skillet. Add the fillets. Cook 3 to 4 minutes on medium heat, then turn and cook 3 to 4 minutes on the other side almost to desired doneness. Remove the meat to individual casserole dishes approximately 5 inches in diameter.
4. Melt the additional butter in the skillet. Add the shallots or onion, mushrooms, and parsley. Cook until the liquid is absorbed.
5. Combine the Dijon mustard, thyme, salt, and pepper with the mushroom mixture. Pour in the broth and the wine. Boil on medium until the liquid is half-reduced. Pour over the meat, dividing it between the two casseroles.
6. Beat the egg whites with a hand blender or mixer until stiff.
7. In a small bowl, beat the yolks with a fork. Fold the egg whites into the yolks. Fold the grated cheese into the egg mixture.
8. Spread the egg mixture in the casseroles, from edge to edge.
9. Place the casseroles in the oven and bake for 20 minutes or until the eggs are a light golden brown. Serve the casseroles on charger plates or hot pads. (Warn diners that dishes are hot to the touch!)

OPTIONS

• Add a 4-ounce can of chicken liver pate to the skillet with the Dijon mustard OR make your own pate. My husband won't even try this. While developing this recipe, 60 chickens arrived for my freezer so I could have made the pate, but I am giving all the livers to our very happy 25 cats!

This recipe is very much like Beef Wellington, only it does not have the carb-filled pastry!

Use an egg separator over a coffeecup; crack the eggs and place in the separator. The whites will flow through the slits into the cup and the yolk will stay in the separator. If necessary, insert a table knife in the slits to loosen the whites.

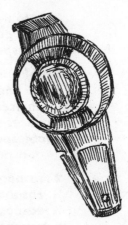

Chapter 2

PORK

Ah, pigs—what can I say? Married to a farmer, I've seen them by the thousands, helped raise them, and even helped chase them back to their pens when they got loose–which usually happened when I was home alone, and usually when I was all cleaned up and ready to go to town. After a job like that, you're dirty right down to the skin, and you smell like. . . well. . . a pig. Now perhaps you have a small inkling why I am grateful that we no longer raise hogs! Although the piglets are awfully cute.

Generally, farmers no longer process their own meat. When it was time for us to butcher a hog, we'd load the selected one into our truck and drive into town. There the butcher would slaughter the pig, skin it, render the lard, carve the carcass into roasts, steaks, and even pork burgers, package each piece, and freeze it all. Then we'd go back to town with boxes to lug the meat to our freezers.

Today's hog is raised to be leaner than ever before. In fact, farmers' pay is docked when they bring fat hogs to market; too much fat, and the hog is rejected. Consequently, the pork available now is high-quality protein; indeed, it is dubbed The Other White Meat.

SAFETY TIPS FOR PORK

• When thawing in the refrigerator, always place the meat on a plate or a pan so that the juices do not contaminate other food. Raw juices often contain bacteria.

PORK STORAGE TIMES

	Refrigerated at 40°F	Frozen at 0°F or colder
Bacon	7 days	1 month
Chops	3 to 5 days	4 to 6 months
Ham, fully cooked, half	3 to 5 days	1 to 2 months
Ham, fully cooked, whole	7 days	1 to 2 months
Ham, fully cooked, sliced	3 to 4 days	1 to 2 months
Hard sausage—pepperoni, jerky sticks	2 to 3 weeks	1 to 2 months
Leftover meat and meat dishes	3 to 4 days	2 to 3 months
Roasts	3 to 5 days	4 to 6 months
Sausage, raw	1 to 2 days	1 to 2 months
Smoked breakfast sausage	7 days	1 to 2 months

INTERNAL COOKED TEMPERATURE FOR PORK

Ham, fresh, raw	160° F
Ham, fully cooked, to reheat	140° F

Pork, all types, including ground.
(Cook until juices run clear.)

Medium	160° F
Well-done	170° F

Never serve pork that has been cooked less than 160° F. Also, always use a meat thermometer. (See Using a Meat Thermometer, p. xviii.)

(Information courtesy of Iowa State University Extension.)

Hickory Smoked Bacon

NO CARBOHYDRATES   **NUMBER OF SERVINGS: AS DESIRED**

1 to 2 pounds bacon
1 tablespoon Camerons hickory chips

1. Place the wood chips in the bottom of a Camerons Stovetop Smoker. Place the drip tray and rack over the chips. Lay the raw bacon on the rack. Slide on the lid, leaving it barely cracked open. Place the Smoker on the largest burner on your stove; turn the heat to medium.
2. As soon as the first wisp of smoke escapes from the Smoker, close the lid and begin timing. Smoking takes 15 minutes; do not overcook.
3. Remove the Smoker from the burner and place on a wire rack. Allow the Smoker to cool for a few minutes. Then remove the bacon.

The bacon is still raw. At this point you can cook it by frying or store it in a tightly closed container in the refrigerator for cooking later.

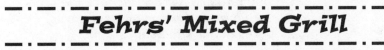

This is fabulous—and so easy! The Smoker does not smoke up your kitchen, although I run my exhaust fan on low anyway. The smoked bacon can be used in many recipes throughout this cookbook.

Fehrs' Mixed Grill

NO CARBOHYDRATES   **NUMBER OF SERVINGS: AS DESIRED**

Bologna sausage
Chicken breasts
Pork Ribletts

1. Preheat the grill on high.
2. Cut all the meat into bite-sized pieces. Place on the grill, close the lid, and reduce the heat. Turn the meat after 5 minutes OR place the meat into a grilling skillet perforated with holes especially made for grilling vegetables. Close the lid and grill as usual. Stir the meat once or twice—this is easier than turning so many pieces on the grill—or if you're skilled, hold the skillet by the handle, toss the meat pieces in the air, and catch them in the skillet.
3. When done, place the meat in an attractive dish and serve.

Brats in Beer

VERY LOW CARBOHYDRATES   **NUMBER OF SERVINGS: 4 OR 5**

2 pounds bratwurst
12-ounce can Miller Lite Beer
1 small onion, sliced

1. Place the sausage in a skillet. Top with the beer and onion. Bring to a boil, reduce the heat, and cover with a lid. Simmer about 20 minutes.
2. Preheat the grill on high.
3. Remove the sausage from the beer and onions and place on grill. Close the lid and reduce the heat. Serve when well-heated and outside is browned.

OPTIONS

- If desired, simmer the sausage in plain water before grilling.
- Serve cooked bratwurst with mustard and diced onion.

Bratwurst is made with raw meat that may not get cooked well enough on the grill. That's why it's safe to simmer on the stove before grilling.

Hot Dogs Smoked with Beer

NO CARBOHYDRATES   **NUMBER OF SERVINGS: AS DESIRED**

Quality no-carb hot dogs (check the label
for no added sugar or other carbs)
2 ounces Miller Lite Beer

1 teaspoon oak wood chips

1. Put the Camerons Stovetop Smoker on the largest burner on your stove. Lay the wood chips in the bottom of the Smoker; place drip tray and rack over the chips. Pour the beer onto the drip tray, then place the hot dogs on the rack. Slide on the lid, leaving it barely cracked. Turn the heat to medium.
2. As soon as the first wisp of smoke escapes from the Smoker, close the lid and begin timing. Cooking takes 15 minutes for 1 pound of hot dogs.

OPTIONS

- Serve the hot dogs with prepared mustard, Westbrae Unsweetened Un-ketchup, and onions.
- If you don't have a Smoker, cook the hot dogs and a few slices of onions in the beer, in a skillet. Cover and steam-cook for a few minutes, then serve.

This is a quick and easy way to cook hot dogs, with a flavor twist. Also, the Smoker cleans easily in the dishwasher.

Back to Protein

Bacon-Cheese Hot Dogs

NO CARBOHYDRATES   **NUMBER OF SERVINGS: AS DESIRED**

Hot dogs, slit lengthwise but not quite to each end
Cheese strips cut to ¼ inch by ¼ inch
Bacon (Check the labels for added sugar)

1. Preheat grill OR broiler OR convection broiler.
2. Stuff the hot dogs with the cheese strips.
3. Wrap the hot dogs with bacon, starting at one end by anchoring the bacon with a toothpick and spiraling to the other end, anchoring with another toothpick. Be certain the hot dog is tightly closed so the cheese will not leak out.
4. Place the hot dogs on the grill OR broiler rack slit side up. Reduce the heat to low and cook until the bacon is done. (If it looks like the cheese won't leak, you can rotate the hot dogs; otherwise leave them slit side up.)
5. Serve—but warn people about the toothpicks!

OPTIONS

• Eliminate the slit and the cheese.   • Serve with Westbrae Unsweetened Un-Ketchup.

Smothered Dogs

VERY LOW CARBOHYDRATES   **NUMBER OF SERVINGS: 3**

1 or 2 tablespoons butter OR olive oil
1 large onion, halved and sliced

1 pound no-carb hot dogs, sliced crosswise
Shredded mozzarella and provolone cheese (optional)

1. Preheat the grill on high.
2. Melt the butter in a cast iron skillet OR coat generously with olive oil.
3. Add onions to the skillet and place the skillet on the grill. Close the lid and reduce the heat to medium. Stirring occasionally, cook onions until they are lightly browned.
4. Add the hot dogs, combine well with the onions. Close the lid and cook until onions are a deep brown and the hot dogs are light brown, stirring occasionally.
5. Remove from the grill, top with cheese if desired, and serve.

OPTIONS

• Cook on the stove in a regular skillet.

Pork   **97**

Eggs & Hot Dogs

VERY LOW CARBOHYDRATES   **NUMBER OF SERVINGS: 3 OR 4**

> *1 tablespoon butter or olive oil*
> *1 pound no-carb hot dogs, cut crosswise in ¼ inch slices*
> *4 hard-boiled eggs, removed from shells and sliced*
> *½ cup chopped tomato, preferably the meaty type like Roma or Beefmaster*
> *2 tablespoons Hellman's Original mayonnaise*
> *2 tablespoons prepared mustard*
> *1 or 2 tablespoons finely diced onion (optional)*

1. Melt the butter in a skillet. Add the hot dogs. Cook until slightly browned.
2. Add the eggs and the tomato. Stir well. Shut off the heat and remove the skillet from the burner.
3. Add the mayonnaise, mustard, and onion to the skillet then serve.

Learn how to hard-boil eggs in the "Hard-boiled Eggs & 2 Butters," p. 256.

Saucy Hot Dogs

LOW CARBOHYDRATES   **NUMBER OF SERVINGS: 3**

> *¼ cup butter*
> *¼ cup finely chopped onion*
> *¼ cup celery*
> *¼ cup green pepper*
>
> *1 pound no-carb hot dogs (check the label for no added sugar), sliced crosswise*
>
> *8 ounce can tomato sauce (no sugar added) OR homemade sauce*
> *1 tablespoon vinegar*
> *1 tablespoon Worcestershire sauce*
> *¼ teaspoon garlic powder*
> *½ of a lemon, thinly sliced, discarding the end piece*

1. Melt the butter in a medium skillet on high heat. Add the onion, celery, and green pepper. Reduce heat to medium and stir fry together.
2. Add the hot dogs and cook until brown, stirring occasionally.
3. Stir in the tomato sauce, vinegar, Worcestershire sauce, and garlic powder. Lay the lemon slices on top of the other ingredients. Cover and cook together for 10 or 15 minutes.
4. Remove the lemon slices, then serve.

OPTIONS
- For a quick supper, serve this dish along with a spoonful of cottage cheese and a green leafy salad.

To prevent spatters on the stovetop, cover the skillet with a spatter screen.

Hot Dogs with Cabbage and Cheese Sauce

VERY LOW CARBOHYDRATES   **NUMBER OF SERVINGS: 3 OR 4**

> **2 cups chopped cabbage (cooks down to 1 cup)**
> **½ cup water**
> **1 pound hot dogs sliced crosswise (check the label for added sugar)**
>
> **⅓ cup heavy cream**
> **1 cup shredded 4-cheese blend: Wisconsin sharp, Vermont white, cheddar and Monterey Jack OR cheeses of choice**

1. Place the cabbage and the water in a skillet. Cover and simmer for 5 minutes, or until the cabbage is tender.
2. Add the hot dog slices. Heat through, uncovered, cooking away all liquid.
3. In a small saucepan, simmer the cream until slightly thickened. Add the cheese, and stir to melt.
4. Pour the cheese sauce over the hot dogs and cabbage. Serve.

Ham Quickie

NO CARBOHYDRATES   **NUMBER OF SERVINGS: AS DESIRED**

> Thick slices of cured ham (check the label
>   for no added sugar)
> Slices of cheddar cheese OR shredded
>   cheddar

1. Top the ham slices with the cheddar cheese. Heat for 30 seconds in the microwave on high. Serve.

> **This couldn't be quicker or easier!**

Ham Hawaiian

VERY LOW CARBOHYDRATES   **NUMBER OF SERVINGS: 1**

> Thick slice of cured ham (check the label for
>   no added sugar)
> 2 tablespoons diced fresh pineapple
> Slices of cheddar cheese OR shredded
>   cheddar

1. Top ham with the pineapple and then the cheddar cheese. Heat for 30 seconds in the microwave on high and serve.

OPTIONS
- Garnish with a single strawberry for a pretty presentation.

> **Avoid canned pineapple in syrup because it is loaded with carbs!**

Baked Ham Steak with Pineapple Mustard Sauce

LOW CARBOHYDRATES   **NUMBER OF SERVINGS:**

> 6-ounce can pineapple juice
> 1 teaspoon whole cloves
> ¼ teaspoon dry mustard
> ½ cup sour cream
>
> 2 to 2½-pound ham steak sliced ½-inch thick

1. In a small saucepan, boil the pineapple juice, clove, and mustard until reduced by half, about 10 or 15 minutes. Remove from the heat and cool completely, then strain out the cloves. Fold in the sour cream. Place in a small serving dish.
2. Preheat the broiler on high. Broil the ham for 5 minutes on each side.
3. Serve the ham—and pass the sauce!

OPTIONS

• The sauce is also wonderful on cured ham slices or pork tenderloins!

This is a fast and easy dish, perfect for company!

Ham & Broccoli Stir Fry

LOW CARBOHYDRATES   NUMBER OF SERVINGS: 2

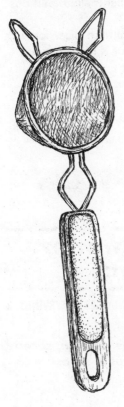

1 tablespoon butter
2 cups diced cured ham
1 to 1½ cups broccoli, cut into bite-sized
*   pieces*
½ to ⅔ cup shredded Colby/Monterey Jack
*   cheese blend OR cheeses of choice*

1. Melt the butter in a skillet, then toss in the ham and broccoli and stir-fry until the ham is lightly browned and the broccoli is bright green.
2. Serve topped with the shredded cheese.

OPTIONS

• Add a few mushrooms with the broccoli.
• Add a few red pepper strips with the broccoli.
• Add a 2-ounce jar of pimento with the broccoli.
• Add ¼ to ½ cup onions in the butter before the ham and broccoli; stir until transparent and browned. Then proceed as above.

This is great when you need something, pronto—only three main ingredients are necessary, and the ham is already cooked.

Ham & Broccoli Cheese Stacks

LOW CARBOHYDRATES   **NUMBER OF SERVINGS: 2**

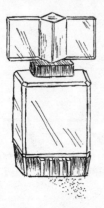

2 thick slices ham
2 tablespoons butter
2 small stalks fresh broccoli, steamed till
    bright green

⅔ cup shredded cheddar, swiss or gouda
    cheese

1. Preheat the broiler on high.
2. Place the ham on oven-safe baking sheet. Put 1
   tablespoon butter on top of each. Put under the
   broiler till meat is hot and butter melted, perhaps
   1 minute.
3. Place one stalk of steamed broccoli on top of each ham slice. Top with
   the cheddar cheese. Put under broiler until cheddar is melted and
   slightly browned.
4. Serve immediately.

OPTIONS

• Cheddar Cheese Sauce: Can make the cheddar into a cheese sauce topping by melting the
⅔ cup cheddar in ¼ cup heavy cream in the microwave. Stir and pour over the broccoli and
ham after heating the ham and butter under the broiler.

> This is really quick and looks attractive, too!

Quick Ham and Summer Squash Skillet

LOW CARBOHYDRATES   **NUMBER OF SERVINGS: 2**

1 tablespoon olive oil
1½ cups fresh young summer squash, sliced
½ medium green pepper, cut in strips
¼ onion, sliced
2 cups cubed cured ham
½ medium tomato
dash freshly ground black pepper (or sub-
    stitute purchased ground black pepper)

dash freshly ground cinnamon (or substitute purchased ground cinnamon)

1. Place the olive oil in a skillet; heat to medium high. Toss in the summer squash, green pepper, and onion and stir fry until lightly browned.
2. Add the cured ham, and continue to stir-fry. Add the tomato and cook it only slightly.
3. Top with the pepper and cinnamon just before serving and stir well.

OPTIONS

- Eliminate the cinnamon. It might seem a strange ingredient here, but don't be put off—it does add a nice flavor to this recipe.

Ham & Bacon Stir Fry

LOW CARBOHYDRATES   **NUMBER OF SERVINGS: 2 OR 3**

2 slices bacon

1 cup diced celery
½ of a medium onion, diced
½ of a medium green pepper, chopped

1 clove garlic, minced
2 cups cubed cured ham

1 tablespoon soy sauce

1. Cook the bacon in a skillet until crisp. Remove from the pan and drain off excess fat.
2. Add the celery, onion, and green pepper to the pan; stir-fry until crisp-tender.
3. Mix in the garlic and ham; heat through.
4. Sprinkle on the crumbled bacon and soy sauce; stir well, and serve.

Ham Stacks with Black Olives

>2 tablespoons Westbrae Unsweetened Un-Ketchup
>1 tablespoon Hellman's Original mayonnaise
>
>2 thick slices cured ham, warmed in a microwave
>4 black olives, sliced
>3 tablespoons finely diced onion OR 2 green onions, including tops
>⅓ cup shredded cheddar/MontereyJjack blend cheeses OR cheeses of choice

1. Preheat the broiler on high.
2. Combine the Un-Ketchup and the mayonnaise. Spread half on each slice of ham.
3. Top with the olives, onion, and cheese.
4. Broil until the cheese is lightly browned then serve.

OPTIONS

• Heat for one minute in the microwave, or until hot.

Ham and Artichokes

>1 tablespoon butter
>2 cups cubed cured ham (check that no sugar was added in processing)
>⅓ to ½ cup canned artichoke hearts, drained and cut into bite-sized pieces (about 7 ounces)
>1 cup shredded cheddar blend cheese

1. Melt the butter in a skillet. Add the ham. Stir-fry for a minute or two until the ham is lightly browned.
2. Add the artichoke hearts and heat through. Divide onto individual serving plates; top with the cheese. If the cheese does not melt, place in the microwave for 20 or 30 seconds on high. Serve.

This is very quick and easy!

Creamed Ham

2 tablespoons butter
⅔ cup chopped onion
3 cups diced cured ham

½ cup sliced black olives
1 cup sour cream

⅓ cup slivered almonds, toasted a few seconds under the broiler (optional)

1. Melt the butter in a skillet; Add the onion and ham, and stir-fry until lightly browned.
2. Add the black olives and the sour cream; stir together until heated through.
3. Top with the toasted almonds and serve.

Although optional, the almonds are a wonderful addition!

Creamed Ham & 3 Cheeses

1 tablespoon butter
2 cups diced cured ham
¼ cup finely chopped onion
2 cloves garlic, minced
½ teaspoon white pepper

1 cup heavy cream

1 cup shredded 4-cheese blend: Wisconsin sharp, Vermont white, Cheddar, and Monterey Jack OR ⅓ cup mozzarella, Parmesan, and Swiss
Minced fresh parsley

1. Melt the butter in a skillet and add the ham, onion, garlic, and white pepper. Stir-fry until the ham and onions are lightly browned.
2. Pour in the cream and simmer until thickened a bit.
3. Add the cheeses and stir until melted. Serve in bowls (this dish will be creamy, like macaroni and cheese). Sprinkle minced parsley on top.

OPTIONS

- Add ¼ cup slivered almonds toasted under the broiler—it's wonderful!
- Add a cup of coarsely chopped fresh broccoli with the ham—also a tasty addition.
- Add 2 or 3 chopped hard-boiled eggs to the sauce OR top each serving with hard-boiled egg slices.

Creamed Ham & Asparagus

LOW CARBOHYDRATES   **NUMBER OF SERVINGS: 2**

1 tablespoon butter
3 to 6 sliced mushrooms, depending on size
*   OR use 4 ounce can sliced mushrooms,*
*   drained*
2 tablespoons finely chopped onion

½ cup heavy cream
2 tablespoons dry white wine

1 egg yolk
3 tablespoons Parmesan cheese

2 thick slices cured ham, heated under the
*   broiler*
8 to 10 asparagus spears, cooked or
*   steamed till bright green*
¼ cup shredded cheddar cheese
Dash paprika

1. Preheat the broiler to high.
2. Melt the butter in a small skillet; saute the mushrooms and onion together.
3. Add the cream and wine to the skillet; simmer on low until thickened.
4. Put a little of the hot cream sauce in a bowl with the egg yolk, stir together, then add the yolk mixture to the skillet. Stir in the Parmesan cheese.
5. Place the ham slices in individual serving casseroles—I use oval French White Corning ware. Top the ham with the asparagus spears. Pour the cream sauce over the asparagus and ham. Top with the shredded cheddar cheese. Sprinkle with a dash of paprika.
6. Place under the broiler until heated through and the cheese is lightly browned.

> **This is wonderful in the spring when I can pick fresh asparagus right outside my kitchen door!**

Ham with Mild Mustard Cream Sauce

LOW CARBOHYDRATES   **NUMBER OF SERVINGS: 4**

1 tablespoon butter
4 thick ham slices

1 cup heavy cream

2 ounce jar pimento
1 teaspoon prepared mustard
½ teaspoon lemon juice

1. Melt the butter in a skillet. Fry the ham on low until lightly browned while you make the sauce.
2. Place the cream in a small saucepan. Simmer without stirring until thickened.
3. Add the lemon juice, pimento, and mustard.
4. Pour the sauce over the heated ham slices and serve.

OPTIONS
• Omit the mustard and lemon juice and add ¼ cup cheddar cheese for Ham with Pimento Cheese Sauce.

Baked Ginger-Wine Ham

LOW CARBOHYDRATES   **NUMBER OF SERVINGS: 5**

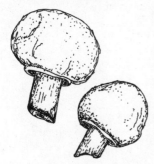

¾ cup white cooking wine
1 tablespoon finely chopped gingerroot
1 ½ teaspoons dry mustard
2 to 2½ pounds cured ham, sliced

1 tablespoon butter
1 small onion, finely chopped
7-ounce can sliced mushrooms, drained

1 cup heavy whipping cream

1. Mix together the white wine, gingerroot, and dry mustard. Pour over the ham slices, cover, and refrigerate for 2 or 3 hours or overnight.
2. Preheat oven to 350°.
3. Remove the ham from the marinade and place in a covered baking dish. Bake for 45 minutes.

4. Melt the butter in a medium skillet. Add the onion and cook until transparent and lightly browned. Add the mushrooms, and heat through.
5. Add the heavy whipping cream and simmer until the sauce is thickened.
6. Serve the ham slices with the mushroom sauce.

Ham & Wilted Spinach

LOW CARBOHYDRATES   **NUMBER OF SERVINGS: 2**

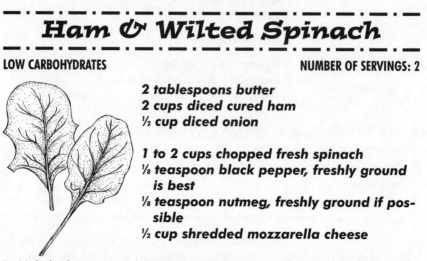

2 tablespoons butter
2 cups diced cured ham
½ cup diced onion

1 to 2 cups chopped fresh spinach
⅛ teaspoon black pepper, freshly ground is best
⅛ teaspoon nutmeg, freshly ground if possible
½ cup shredded mozzarella cheese

1. Melt the butter in a skillet and add the ham and onion. Saute on medium until the onion is transparent.
2. Toss in the spinach, pepper, and nutmeg, stir constantly until the spinach is wilted.
3. Just before serving, top with the shredded mozzarella cheese.

OPTIONS
• Four ounces of sliced mushrooms can be added to the ham and onion.

Ham with Mushroom Sauce

VERY LOW CARBOHYDRATES　　　　　　　　**NUMBER OF SERVINGS: 6**

> **2 pounds cured ham, about 10 slices (check the label for no added sugar)**
> **8 ounces sliced mushrooms**
> **2 tablespoons butter**
> **1 cup heavy cream**
> **1 tablespoon cooking sherry**
> **2 tablespoons finely chopped fresh parsley**
> **Additional parsley as garnish**

1. Place the ham in a 350° oven in a covered dish while you prepare the sauce.
2. Melt the butter in a skillet and saute the mushrooms. Add the cream and allow to simmer, without stirring, until thickened. Stir in the sherry and parsley.
3. Place the warm ham slices on a serving platter; pour the sauce over all. Garnish with additional parsley sprigs, and serve immediately.

Basic Ham Salad

TRACE OR VERY LOW CARBOHYDRATES　　　　　**NUMBER OF SERVINGS: 2**

> **2 cups diced cured ham (¼-inch cubes), about 8 ounces**
> **¼ cup Hellman's Original mayonnaise**
> **2 tablespoons Dijon mustard**
> **½ teaspoon dried savory leaves**
>
> **Lettuce**
> **Slice of sweet red pepper or red radish for garnish, (optional)**

Combine all of the ingredients and serve on a lettuce bed. Garnish, if desired, and serve.

OPTIONS

- Substitute Worcestershire sauce for the Dijon mustard.
- Add ½ cup shredded cheddar cheese and increase the mayonnaise to ⅓ cup.
- Add 3 chopped green onions, including tops.
- Top with hard-boiled egg slices.

> **This is quick, easy, and outstanding!**

Pork　　　　　　　　　　　　　　　　　　**109**

Ham & Artichoke Salad

2 cups cubed cured ham
⅓ cup sliced canned artichoke hearts,
   drained
6 large black olives, sliced
¼ cup chopped green pepper
¼ cup grated Parmesan cheese
¼ cup chopped onion
1 tablespoon finely minced fresh parsley
½ teaspoon purchased Italian spice blend
2 tablespoons olive oil
2 tablespoons red wine vinegar

Lettuce
Tomato slices

1. In a medium bowl, mix the ham with all of the ingredients except the lettuce. If there is time, chill for a few hours—but you can eat it immediately.
2. Serve on a bed of lettuce garnished with a thin slice of tomato.

Ham and Peach Salad

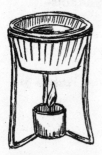

2 cups cured ham
1 small fresh or canned peach in natural
   juices, diced
¼ cup Hellman's Original mayonnaise
Gingerroot, ¼-inch slice ½-inch in diameter,
   finely chopped

Lettuce OR spinach leaf
Dash paprika OR cinnamon

1. Combine the ham, peach, mayonnaise and gingerroot.
2. Serve on a lettuce bed or spinach leaf topped with a sprinkle of paprika or cinnamon.

OPTIONS
- Substitute ⅓ cup of mandarin oranges, drained, for the peach.
- Instead of ham, cooked chicken, pork, or tuna works well.

Back to Protein

Pork Chops with Herb Butter

NO CARBOHYDRATES   **NUMBER OF SERVINGS: 2**

> 2 pork chops, butterfly or loin
>
> 2 tablespoons butter, softened to room temperature
> ½ teaspoon crushed rosemary (use a mortar and pestle)
> ¼ teaspoon sage
> Salt and pepper to taste

1. Broil, grill, or pan-fry the chops in butter until done. If broiling or grilling, rub olive oil into both sides of the meat to keep moist.
2. Blend together the butter and herbs. Serve half on each chop.

OPTIONS

- Melt the butter in the microwave on high for 10 seconds, add the herbs, and pour over the chops. Or melt the butter mixture in individual ceramic butter warmers, with a chafing candle lit underneath. Diners can dip bite-sized pieces of pork into the butter.

Grilled Herb Pork Chops

VERY LOW CARBOHYDRATES   **NUMBER OF SERVINGS: 2**

> 1 tablespoon olive oil
> 2 cloves garlic, minced
> ½ tablespoon crushed rosemary
> 4 teaspoons dried parsley flakes OR 2 tablespoons fresh minced parsley
>
> 2 pounds Iowa Chops OR pork loin chops
> Parsley for garnish (optional)

1. Preheat the grill on high.
2. Combine the olive oil, garlic, rosemary, and parsley in a coffeecup. Rub thoroughly into both sides of the chops.
3. Place the chops on the grill and reduce the heat to low. Close the lid and cook until done—when the meat inside is opaque and no longer pink. Turn once half way through cooking.
4. Serve garnished with parsley sprigs, if desired.

Pork Chops with Homemade Pork Seasoning

TRACE CARBOHYDRATES

NUMBER OF SERVINGS:

Iowa Chops OR pork loin chops
Pork Seasoning (recipe follows)

1. Preheat the grill to high.
   To make seasoning, combine the following in a small jar:

   3 tablespoons paprika
   1 tablespoon celery salt
   2 teaspoons ground coriander
   1 teaspoon chili powder
   1 teaspoon cayenne
   ½ teaspoon ground nutmeg

2. Sprinkle the seasoning on both sides of the pork chops.
3. Place the chops on the grill, close the lid and reduce the heat to medium. Cook to desired doneness, turning occasionally, and serve. Reserve extra seasoning for future use.

> **Save empty shake-top spice jars for homemade seasoning mixes. Tape a label on the front to identify the blend for future use.**

Bob's Favorite Pork Chops

VERY LOW CARBOHYDRATES

NUMBER OF SERVINGS: 2 OR 3

1 to 1½ pounds of pork chops (2 or 3)
½ cup no-carb soy sauce

5 to 6 cloves of minced garlic
Gingerroot 1 inch in diameter by ½ inch long, very finely chopped

1. Combine the meat in the soy, garlic and gingerroot mixture in a plastic bag or covered container. Refrigerate from 4 to 24 hours; turn once or twice.
2. Preheat the grill on high.
3. Coat the grill rack with vegetable oil spray, immediately place the chops on the grill. Turn the heat down to medium and cook to desired doneness. Serve.

Barb's Favorite Pork Chops

VERY LOW CARBOHYDRATES   **NUMBER OF SERVINGS: 2 OR 3**

1 to 1½ pounds pork chops (2 or 3)
1 tablespoon butter

½ cup chicken broth (homemade or canned)
      OR ½ cup water plus 1 teaspoon chicken
      bouillon granules
¼ cup finely chopped green pepper
¼ cup finely chopped celery (one rib)
2 tablespoons pineapple juice
1½ teaspoons apple vinegar (or white vinegar)
½ teaspoon soy sauce
¼ teaspoon Worcestershire sauce
⅛ teaspoon ground mustard

1. Trim any excess fat from the chops.
2. Melt the butter in a skillet and fry the pork chops until browned on both sides.
3. In a 2-cup measure, combine the rest of the other ingredients. Add the mixture to the skillet and simmer, covered, on medium low for 10 minutes. Turn chops over and continue simmering, uncovered, until the liquid is reduced by half, about 10 more minutes. Serve.

OPTIONS

• Add ¼ teaspoon freshly grated gingerroot to the broth mixture before cooking.

Pork Chops in White Wine

1 pound pork chops (butterfly or loin)
1½ teaspoons bacon drippings (saved from breakfast) OR butter
Freshly ground black pepper to taste
½ cup white cooking wine plus 1 teaspoon instant chicken bouillon granules
1 medium onion, sliced

1. In a skillet, brown the chops on both sides in bacon drippings.
2. Cover the chops with onion slices. Add the white wine, black pepper and chicken bouillon. Simmer 30 minutes covered, then uncover and simmer another 10 or 15 minutes until the liquid is nearly gone. Scrape the bottom to loosen any browned bits to incorporate them into the onions. Serve.

OPTIONS

• You don't have to double the wine if you're doubling the recipe. For every additional ½ pound pork chop, add 2 tablespoons more wine plus ¼ teaspoon more chicken bouillon.
• Another favorite method of cooking this is to brown the chops, then remove them from the skillet. Add another tablespoon of butter or olive oil and the onion slices, and stir-fry on medium-high heat until well-browned. Then add the wine and bouillon and simmer, uncovered, scraping the bottom of the skillet to loosen all the browned bits. Serve this over the pork chops. Delicious!

Baked Chili Chops

1 pound pork tenderloin, cut into ¾ inch slices, OR butterfly chops OR regular pork chops

1 tablespoon Westbrae Unsweetened Un-Ketchup
Chili powder, as desired
2 onion slices, cut to 1½-inch thick
1 whole lemon, cut in ¼ inch slices. (Do not use the ends of the lemons because the white pith turns bitter in cooking.)

1. Preheat oven to 350°.
2. Place the meat in a single layer in a baking dish just large enough to hold them.
3. Brush the Un-Ketchup over the tops of the meat. Sprinkle chili powder over the chops.
4. Top with the onion slices; top the onions with the lemon slices.
5. Cover and bake for 30 minutes at 350°, then uncover and bake another 20 to 30 minutes. Remove the lemon slices and serve.

OPTIONS
- Made this on the stove by simmering on medium low heat for 30 minutes, uncovering and then continuing to simmer another 30 minutes.

"Breaded" Pork Chops

NO CARBOHYDRATES   **NUMBER OF SERVINGS: 2**

2 Pork chops, butterfly or regular, with or without bone

1 egg

1 cup finely ground pork rinds

1. Preheat the oven to 350° or a convection oven to 325°.
2. Beat the egg in a coffeecup with a fork until the yolk is blended.
3. Put the egg in one pan (a small pieplate works fine) and the ground pork rinds in another. Dip both sides of each chop first in the egg and then in the rinds. Discard all leftover pork rinds that you've used for dipping.
4. Place a rack in an ovensafe pan; spray the rack and the pan with a vegetable coating. Lay coated meat on the rack.
5. Bake for 30 to 40 minutes (or convection oven bake for 20 to 30 minutes), depending on the thickness of the chops, until done. Serve.

OPTIONS
- This can be pan-fried after step 3. Omit step 1 and use 1 tablespoon oil or butter per chop. Fry one side till browned, then turn and fry the other side until the meat is done.

The egg and ground-up pork rinds make a crust so the meat is tender and juicy.

Chops in Beer

1 pound pork chops or butterfly chops
1 to 2 tablespoons butter or olive oil

1 medium onion, sliced
½ cup Miller Lite Beer plus ¼ teaspoon of
  beef bouillon granules OR ¼ teaspoon
  Beefer Upper

1. Melt the butter in a skillet and fry the chops until well-browned on both sides.
2. Remove the chops to a small skillet and place on another burner on the lowest temperature to keep meat warm.
3. Put onion rings in first skillet and brown on medium high heat.
4. Add the beer and beef flavoring to the onions, simmer till liquid is reduced by half, stirring to loosen the brown coating on the skillet, which makes a nice sauce.
5. Serve the chops topped with the onion sauce.

Easy Wine-Italian Pork Loin Chops

¾ cup low-carb Italian salad dressing (see
  also recipe for homemade Italian dress-
  ing on page 296)
¾ cup dry red wine

1½ pounds pork loin chops

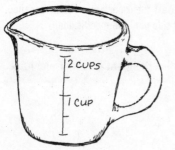

1. Combine salad dressing and wine; stir.
2. Pour marinade over pork, turning to coat all sides. Cover and refrigerate about 2 to 4 hours.
3. Preheat grill on high.
4. Remove pork from marinade and place on grill. Close lid and reduce temperature to medium or low. Watch closely to prevent burning or flare-ups. Turn chops once or twice. Cook to desired doneness and serve.

Pork Chops Parmesan

2 tablespoons butter
1 teaspoon paprika
¾ teaspoon garlic powder
½ teaspoon thyme
¼ teaspoon black pepper

1 pound pork tenderloin or loin chops
1 to 2 tablespoons grated Parmesan cheese

1. Preheat the grill on high.
2. Place the butter in a 1-cup measuring glass; microwave on high for 30 seconds or until softened.
3. Add the paprika, garlic, thyme, and black pepper to the butter to make a paste.
4. Use a narrow rubber scraper to divide the paste and coat each pork chop. Top with the Parmesan cheese.
5. Place the pork on the grill with the paste side up. Turn the heat down to medium, (about 350°). Close the lid and grill for about 15 to 20 minutes. Watch carefully, the last 5 minutes because you will not turn the chops over and you want the bottoms to be browned, but not blackened. Serve.

OPTIONS

• Although I prefer not turning the chops as they cook (this allows the butter and herbs to better penetrate the meat), you can grill the chops for 10 minutes, turn them over, apply the butter paste, and then grill for another 5 to 10 minutes.

• If the weather doesn't permit grilling, bake or convection oven bake at 350° in a cast-iron skillet generously coated with 2 to 3 tablespoons of olive oil. Do not cover, and do not turn the meat. It will take about the same amount of time.

> **If your cast iron skillet has a wooden handle, remove it before placing the pan on the grill or in the oven.**

Barbecued Pork Chops

VERY LOW CARBOHYDRATES   **NUMBER OF SERVINGS: 4**

2 tablespoons butter
1½ to 2 pounds pork tenderloin OR loin
  chops OR butterfly chops

½ cup Westbrae Unsweetened Un-Ketchup
2 tablespoons vinegar
½ teaspoon celery seed
¼ teaspoon nutmeg
1 bay leaf

1. Preheat the oven to bake at 350° OR convection bake at 325°.
2. Melt the butter in a skillet and brown both sides of the pork. Place the meat snugly in a single layer in a covered ovenproof casserole.
3. Combine the Un-Ketchup, vinegar, celery seed, nutmeg and bay leaf. Spread over the pork and cover. Oven bake for 50 minutes, then remove the lid and bake OR convection bake another 15 minutes, adding a little water if it looks dry. Serve.

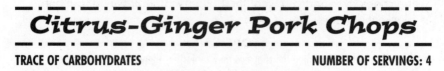

The meat turns out nice and tender.

Citrus-Ginger Pork Chops

TRACE OF CARBOHYDRATES   **NUMBER OF SERVINGS: 4**

1 tablespoon soy sauce
1 tablespoon water
¾ teaspoon minced gingerroot OR ¼ teaspoon ginger
¼ teaspoon orange zest

2 pounds Iowa Chops OR pork loin chops
Orange slices for garnish (optional)

1. Preheat the grill on high.
2. Combine the soy sauce, water, gingerroot and orange zest in a coffeecup.
3. Place the chops on the grill and reduce the heat to medium. Close the lid and cook until done—when the meat inside is opaque and no longer pink; turn once halfway through cooking.
4. About 5 minutes before serving, brush the gingerroot mixture on top of the chops.
5. Serve garnished with thin orange slices, if desired.

Basic Stovetop Pork Tenderloin

NO CARBOHYDRATES   **NUMBER OF SERVINGS: 2**

1 to 2 tablespoons butter
1 pound pork tenderloin
Salt and pepper as desired

⅓ cup water OR broth OR wine

1. Melt the butter in a skillet, add the pork, and saute on medium heat until done and both sides are browned.
2. Add the water, broth, or wine and simmer on the lowest setting. Scrape up the browned bits on the bottom of the skillet while the liquid is being reduced.
3. Serve the meat with any remaining liquid on top.

OPTIONS
• Add a few sliced mushrooms to the skillet before adding the liquid.
• Add a few onion slices to the skillet before adding the liquid.
• Add ¼ teaspoon dried herb or herb combination of your choice to the liquid—try dry mustard, garlic powder, sage and/or thyme.

Basic Grilled Pork Tenderloin

LOW CARBOHYDRATES   **NUMBER OF SERVINGS: 2**

1 pound pork tenderloin, cut into 4, 1-inch slices

1½ teaspoons dry mustard
½ teaspoon garlic powder
½ teaspoon salt

1. Preheat the grill on high.
2. Combine the mustard, garlic powder, and salt; rub into both sides of the pork.
3. Let the meat sit awhile if you have time. Otherwise, place the meat on the grill. Close the lid and reduce the heat to medium. After about 10 minutes, when the bottom is browned, turn the meat. Cook until done. Serve.

Grilled Pork Tenderloin with Bacon and Onions

Pork tenderloin for two servings, about 1 pound, sliced 1 to 1¼ inches thick (or cut your own from a whole tenderloin)

4 slices of bacon (check label for no added sugar)

2 slices of onion

salt and pepper to taste

2 slices tomato cut about ¼ inch thick (Beefmaster variety is ideal)

2 slices cheese of choice (mozzarella, Swiss, American)

1. Heat the grill on high.
2. Trim the excess fat from the tenderloins. If the cuts are small, put two together for each serving.
3. Criss-cross 2 pieces of bacon in an X-shape, and top the bacon with one slice of onion, then place a piece of pork on top of onion. Bring the ends of bacon up and over the top of each piece of pork. Secure with a toothpick.
4. Grill on low to medium heat, turning often with tongs, for about 45 minutes or until nearly done. (On our Weber gas grill, we turn off the middle burner and run the outer burners on low.)
5. Top each tenderloin with a slice of tomato and grill another 10 minutes.
6. Top each tomato with a slice of cheese and leave on the grill another minute or so, until the cheese is partly melted. Remove the toothpicks and serve.

OPTIONS

• Hickory-smoked bacon is wonderful in this recipe. Smoke your own. See recipe on page 95.

Hickory Smoked Pork Tenderloins

NO CARBOHYDRATES   **NUMBER OF SERVINGS: 2**

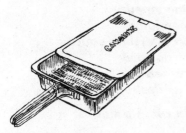

1 tablespoon olive oil
¼ teaspoon dry thyme
1 pound pork tenderloin OR loin chops
1 teaspoon Camerons hickory wood chips

1. Combine the olive oil and thyme and rub over the pork.
2. Place the wood chips in the bottom of a Camerons Stovetop Smoker; place the drip tray and rack over the chips. Lay the meat on the rack. Slide on the lid, leaving it barely cracked. Place the Smoker on the largest burner on your stove; turn the heat to medium.
3. As soon as the first wisp of smoke escapes from the Smoker, close the lid and begin timing. Cooking takes 25 minutes. Remove the smoker from the burner and serve the meat.

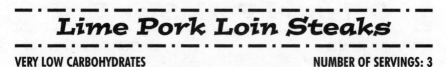

Lime Pork Loin Steaks

VERY LOW CARBOHYDRATES   **NUMBER OF SERVINGS: 3**

¼ cup red cooking wine
2 tablespoons olive oil
2 tablespoons lime juice (can use Real Lime)
1 tablespoon dried minced onion
1 teaspoon thyme
½ teaspoon marjoram
1 bay leaf, crushed
1½ pounds pork tenderloin, cut into 3 steaks, OR 3 pork loin chops

1. Mix together all of the ingredients except the meat. Pour over the pork and marinate overnight or all day in the refrigerator.
2. Grill to desired doneness.

OPTIONS
• Try cooking this in the Cameron's stovetop smoker.

Pork

Marinated Pork Loin

VERY LOW CARBOHYDRATES   **NUMBER OF SERVINGS: 2**

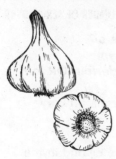

¼ **cup olive oil**
3 **tablespoons soy sauce**
2 **tablespoons wine vinegar**
1 **tablespoon lemon juice**
1 **tablespoon Worcestershire sauce**
1½ **teaspoons dry mustard**
1 **clove garlic, crushed**
Salt and pepper as desired

1 **pound pork loin cut into steaks**

1. Combine all of the ingredients except the pork.
2. Place the pork in a plastic bag and pour the marinade over the meat. Turn the pork to coat all sides. Close bag and refrigerate for 1 to 2 hours.
3. Preheat the grill on high.
4. Place the pork on the grill and close the lid. Reduce the heat to low-medium and cook until done, turning about halfway through. Remove from the grill and serve.

Oriental Pork Stir Fry

LOW CARBOHYDRATES   **NUMBER OF SERVINGS: 2 OR 3**

1 **pound pork loin, cut into bite-sized cubes**
1 **tablespoon no carb soy sauce (check that it doesn't have added sugar)**
1 **tablespoon vinegar**

1 **teaspoon sesame oil**
½ **teaspoon ginger OR** ¼ **teaspoon grated gingerroot**
1 **clove garlic, minced**

2 **tablespoons olive oil**

¾ **cup sliced bamboo shoots**
4 **ounces mushrooms, sliced**
½ **of a green pepper, cut into strips**

1. Mix together the pork, soy sauce, vinegar, sesame oil, ginger, and garlic.

2. Heat a skillet or wok on high. Add the olive oil. Stir-fry the pork mixture for 3 to 4 minutes, or until pork is nearly done.
3. Add the vegetables. Cook until the meat is done and the vegetables are crisp-tender. Serve.

OPTIONS

• You have great leeway on this recipe's vegetables. Just add 1 to 2 cups of any combination of the following: celery, water chestnuts (use only a few), green pepper, mushrooms, onions, etc.
• Some people like to sprinkle no-carb soy sauce on top of their serving.

Quick Cabbage & Pork Stir Fry

LOW CARBOHYDRATES   **NUMBER OF SERVINGS: 2 OR 3**

2 tablespoons olive oil
1 pound pork loin, cut into bite sized cubes

1 small carrot sliced (or ½ of a large carrot)

1 teaspoon ginger powder
2 cups fresh cabbage, very coarsely chopped

Soy sauce (optional)

1. Stir-fry the pork in the olive oil in a skillet or wok.
2. Add the carrots and ginger and stir-fry until the carrot is tender and the meat is done.
3. Mix in the cabbage and stir-fry just until wilted and brighter. Serve with soy sauce, if desired.

OPTIONS

• About ½ cup chopped onions can be added with the carrot.

Colorful Pork Stir Fry

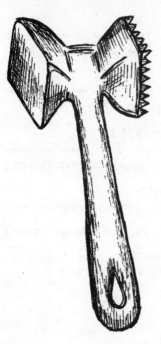

1 pound lean pork cut into 1-inch cubes (I use loin)
2 tablespoons no-carb soy sauce
2 tablespoons dry white wine
¼ to ½ teaspoon grated gingerroot

1 small carrot, cut into thin strips
½ red sweet pepper, cut into thin slices
4 ounces fresh mushrooms, sliced
¼ cup chopped onions

1 or 2 tablespoons olive oil

1. Stir together the pork, soy sauce, wine, and gingerroot. Allow to marinate while you chop the vegetables.
2. Heat the olive oil in a wok or skillet. Toss in the pork mixture and stir-fry for 3 minutes on high, stirring constantly.
3. Add the vegetables and stir-fry until the meat is done and the vegetables are crisp-tender about 5 more minutes on high.

OPTIONS

• Serve with soy sauce, as desired.

"Breaded" Pork Tenderloins

NO CARBOHYDRATES NUMBER OF SERVINGS: 2

About 1 pound pork tenderloin
1 egg
¾ cup ground pork rinds

¼ teaspoon rosemary, crushed
⅛ teaspoon pepper

1. Preheat the oven to 400°.
2. Cut the tenderloin lengthwise, in half, almost all the way through. Use

the flat side of a mallet to pound the meat to ¼ inch thickness.

3. Beat the egg with a fork until the yolk is blended.
4. Combine the pork rinds, rosemary, and pepper in a pie plate; blend well.
5. Dip each piece of meat into the egg and then into the rind mixture, coating both sides. (Note: Discard any leftover rind.)
6. Place on a broiler pan rack, sprayed with vegetable oil. Bake for 30 minutes, or until the meat is done and the coating is lightly browned.
7. Remove and serve hot.

OPTIONS

• Substitute ⅓ cup buttermilk for the egg.
• Drizzle 2 to 3 tablespoons of melted butter on top of the pork-rind coating before baking the tenderloins—wonderful!

Applesauce-Baked Pork Tenderloin

LOW CARBOHYDRATES   **NUMBER OF SERVINGS: 8**

8 pork tenderloin steaks cut about 1 inch thick (about 4 pounds)
2 tablespoons butter or olive oil

2 large cloves minced garlic
2 teaspoons minced gingerroot
½ cup rose wine
¼ cup no carb soy sauce
1 pound can low-carb applesauce (Musselman's Natural has 39 grams total carb)

1. Preheat oven on bake at 350° OR convection bake at 325°.
4. Brown the steaks on both sides in a skillet in melted butter or olive oil. Transfer the steaks to a casserole dish, lined to a single thickness.
5. Brown the garlic and gingerroot in the skillet. Turn off the heat and pour in the wine, stirring and scraping the bottom of the pan to loosen browned bits. Stir in the soy sauce and the applesauce. Pour the mixture over the tenderloin.
6. Bake, uncovered, for 1 hour OR convection bake, uncovered, about 45 minutes. Serve.

> **This recipe is great for a dinner party!**

Pork Tenderloin with Mushroom and Tomato Cream Sauce

LOW CARBOHYDRATES   **NUMBER OF SERVINGS: 4**

2 tablespoons butter
3 shallot cloves, chopped
1 large garlic clove, minced
8 ounces sliced mushrooms

1½ to 2 pounds pork tenderloin, cut into
    bite-sized chunks
½ cup white cooking wine

1 cup canned chopped tomatoes, drained
½ cup heavy whipping cream
½ teaspoon allspice
½ teaspoon basil
¼ teaspoon thyme
salt and pepper to taste

1. Melt the butter in a large skillet and add the shallot, garlic, and mushrooms. Stir-fry on medium-high heat about 2 to 3 minutes.
2. Lower the heat to medium and add the pork, cooking about 6 to 7 minutes, until nearly done.
3. Turn the heat to medium-high and add the wine, stirring to loosen the browned bits on the bottom of the pan.
4. Add the tomatoes, cream, allspice, basil, thyme, salt, and pepper and stir. Simmer on low until sauce is thickened, about 10 to 15 minutes. Serve.

OPTIONS
• Substitute 2 medium fresh tomatoes for the canned tomatoes; peel, seed, and cut into bite-sized pieces.

Pork Tenderloin in Mushroom-Beer Sauce

LOW CARBOHYDRATES   **NUMBER OF SERVINGS: 2**

1 tablespoon butter
1 pound pork tenderloin cut into fillets
¼ cup finely diced onion
1 garlic clove, minced

1 cup sliced mushrooms (about 4 ounces)
¼ teaspoon thyme

About 1 cup Miller Lite Beer (about 8 ounces)
1 tablespoon fresh minced parsley

1. Melt the butter in a medium skillet; add the pork and cook until lightly browned on both sides. Remove from the skillet and keep warm.
4. Add the onion and garlic to the skillet; saute together about 2 minutes.
5. Add the mushrooms and thyme and cook about 3 minutes.
6. Return the meat to the skillet. Add enough beer to cover the meat. Bring to a boil then and reduce the heat to simmer on low for about 45 minutes. The liquid will be largely evaporated.
7. Sprinkle parsley on top and serve.

Mom's Pork Roast

NO OR VERY LOW CARBOHYDRATES　　　**NUMBER OF SERVINGS: AS DESIRED**

1 or 2 tablespoons butter
1 pork roast
Sage
Salt and pepper
Sliced onions (optional)
Water

1. Preheat the oven to 350°.
6. Melt the butter in a skillet on medium-high heat. Fry the roast in the butter, turning to brown all sides.
7. Place roast in a covered roasting pan. Sprinkle with sage, salt, and pepper. Place the sliced onions over the roast. Pour a little water in the bottom of the roaster, perhaps 1 cup. Cover and bake.
8. Let the covered roaster sit on the counter for about 10 minutes. Slice and serve.

Loin Roast with Bacon

VERY LOW CARBOHYDRATES   **NUMBER OF SERVINGS: 6**

4 pound pork loin roast
½ teaspoon ginger
¼ teaspoon garlic powder
¼ teaspoon pepper
1 medium onion, chopped
¼ to ½ cup water (enough to coat the bottom of the pan)

3 or 4 slices of bacon, fried crisp and crumbled
Drippings from roast
1 cup beef broth
1/2 cup sherry cooking wine

1. Preheat the oven to 325°.
2. Place the meat in a covered roasting pan. Sprinkle with the ginger, garlic, and pepper and top with the chopped onion. Pour in the water. Cover and bake for about 3 hours. Add a little more water while cooking if necessary.
3. Just before serving, fry the bacon in a skillet and remove to a paper towel. Drain off all the grease.
4. Pour the roast drippings and the beef broth into the skillet and simmer 3 minutes. Remove from the heat. Add the crumbled bacon and sherry and serve as a sauce with the roast pork.

Let the roast stand on the counter for about 15 minutes before slicing.

Paprika-Ginger Pork Roast

TRACE CARBOHYDRATES   **NUMBER OF SERVINGS: 8**

1 teaspoon black pepper
1 teaspoon paprika
1 teaspoon garlic powder
1 teaspoon dry ginger
Salt to taste
4-pound pork loin roast

1. Preheat the oven to 350° or a convection oven to 325°.

2. Mix the pepper, paprika, garlic powder, ginger, and salt together; sprinkle all over the roast and then rub in.
3. Place on a rack in a roasting pan and bake, covered, about 2 hours OR convection bake, uncovered, about 1 ½ hours.

OPTIONS
Use 2 cloves of garlic and 1-inch diameter by ¼-inch slice of fresh gingerroot instead of the dry; rub into the roast before sprinkling on the pepper and paprika.

Pork Loin Roast with Sour Cream Sauce

VERY LOW CARBOHYDRATES   **NUMBER OF SERVINGS: 4**

2-pound boneless pork loin roast

½ cup sour cream
¼ cup grated Parmesan cheese
1 tablespoon olive oil
1 tablespoon lemon juice
1 teaspoon Dijon mustard
½ teaspoon dried dill weed
½ teaspoon salt, or as desired
¼ teaspoon pepper, or as desired

1. Trim the excess fat from the roast. Butterfly the meat by cutting in half parallel to the surface of the meat, but do not cut all the way through. Open at the cut and lie flat in a small roasting pan with a lid.
2. Combine the remaining ingredients and spread over the roast. Cover and refrigerate for 2 hours to marinate, if you have the time.
3. Preheat oven to 350°.
4. Bake, covered for 90 minutes, or until done (the meat thermometer reads 170°).
5. Let rest, cover for 10 minutes, then slice and serve.

Ginger-Mustard Marinated Pork Roast

TRACE CARBOHYDRATES   **NUMBER OF SERVINGS: 6 TO 8**

½ cup soy sauce
½ cup sherry cooking wine
1 tablespoon dry mustard
1 teaspoon minced gingerroot
1 teaspoon thyme

2 cloves garlic, minced

4 to 5 pound pork roast

1. Combine all of the ingredients except the meat; mix well.
2. Place the pork in a large plastic bag; pour in the marinade. Work the air out of the bag and close tightly. Refrigerate 2 hours or overnight, turning the roast once in a while if convenient.
3. Preheat the oven to 350° OR a convection oven to 325°.
4. Remove the roast from the marinade and place on a rack in a roasting pan.
5. Bake, uncovered, for 2½ to 3 hours OR convection bake 2 to 2¼ hours, or until done.
6. Let rest on the counter 10 minutes; slice and serve.

Sesame Pork Roast

VERY LOW CARBOHYDRATES   **NUMBER OF SERVINGS: 2**

2-pound pork loin roast, trimmed of excess fat

½ cup soy sauce
2 tablespoons Westbrae Unsweetened Un-Ketchup
2 cloves garlic, minced

3 tablespoons sesame seeds
Prepared mustard

1. Place the roast in a plastic bag.
2. Combine the soy sauce, Un-Ketchup, and garlic. Pour over the roast. Squeeze the air out of the bag and seal tightly. Turn the bag to coat all sides of the meat with the marinade. Refrigerate for 2 to 24 hours.
3. Preheat the oven to bake OR convection bake at 325°.
4. Place the roast on a rack in a roasting pan, uncovered. Bake for 60 minutes OR convection bake for 50 minutes, or until the thermometer reads 160°.
5. Top the roast with sesame seeds; return to the oven for another 5 minutes. Slice and serve with mustard, if desired.

OPTIONS
• This recipe is quite delicious without the sesame seeds and mustard.

Chapter 3

LAMB

Although many farmers in our area raise sheep, few of us eat it and many have never even cooked with it! It's only occasionally available in local stores, often by special request. The farmers I interviewed said their lamb meat was shipped out of the Midwest. But the butcher at our local store was most helpful in providing me with lamb and advice.

SAFETY TIPS FOR LAMB

• Do not store fresh lamb for more than 3 days in the refrigerator—freeze it.

• When thawing in the refrigerator, always place the meat on a plate or a pan so that juices do not contaminate other food. Raw juices often contain bacteria.

COOKING LAMB

Less tender cuts, shank crosscuts, or chuck generally require moist heat (with added liquid), such as braising and cooking in liquid/stewing. Tender lamb cuts from the breast, rack, loin, sirloin, and leg can be cooked with dry heat (no added liquid), such as by roasting, broiling, grilling, pan-broiling, and pan-frying. Lamb can be roasted rare, medium, or well-done.

• For medium-rare, the thermometer should read 145 to 150° and the meat should be reddish inside.

• For medium, the thermometer should read 160° and the meat should be brownish-pink inside.

• For well-done, the thermometer should read 170° and there should be no pink inside.

HOW TO ROAST LAMB

• Place the lamb, fat side up (if present), on a rack in an open, shallow roasting pan.

• Rub with seasonings, if desired.

• Insert the meat thermometer into the center of the thickest muscle of the meat.

• Do not add water or liquid, and do not cover.

• Roast at 325° F until the meat thermometer registers 5° below desired doneness.

• Remove from the oven, cover with foil, and let stand 15 to 20 minutes before slicing. Smaller roasts should stand 5 to 10 minutes before carving.

LAMB STORAGE TIMES

	Refrigerated at 40°F	Frozen at 0°F or colder
Cooked lamb	3 to 4 days	2 to 3 months
Ground lamb	1 to 2 days	3 to 4 months
Roasts and chops	2 to 3 days	6 to 9 months

(Information courtesy of the American Lamb Council.)

With the exception of the Curry Lamb Stew, the following lamb recipes are from the American Lamb Council, or adapted from Council recipes.

Back to Protein

Grilled Lamb Steak with 3 Sauces

VERY LOW CARBOHYDRATES   **NUMBER OF SERVINGS: 2**

> **2 lamb center round leg steaks, cut ¾-inch thick**
> **Basting sauce (see below)**

1. Preheat the grill on high heat.
2. Trim any fat from the steaks.
3. Place the steaks on the grill and reduce the heat to medium. Grill 8 to 10 minutes to desired doneness, turning once and occasionally brushing with desired basting sauce.
4. Remove from grill and serve.

Mint Raspberry Sauce:
> 2 tablespoons olive oil
> 2 tablespoons raspberry vinegar
> 1 teaspoon chopped fresh mint
> 1 clove garlic, minced

Curry Sauce:
> ¼ cup sour cream
> 1 teaspoon curry powder
> 1 clove garlic, minced

Lemon Pepper Sauce:
> 2 tablespoons olive oil
> 1 tablespoon red wine vinegar
> 1 tablespoon finely chopped onion
> 1½ teaspoons lemon pepper

Herbed Grilled Lamb Steaks

VERY LOW CARBOHYDRATES   **NUMBER OF SERVINGS: 2 OR 3**

> **¼ cup lemon juice**
> **¼ cup olive oil**
> **1 teaspoon basil**
> **1 teaspoon salt**
> **½ teaspoon paprika**
> **½ teaspoon onion powder**
> **¼ teaspoon garlic powder**
>
> **2 or 3 lamb leg steaks, cut 1-inch thick**

1. Combine all the marinade ingredients except the meat and pour over the lamb. Cover and refrigerate for 2 to 24 hours.
2. Preheat the grill.
3. Remove the meat from the marinade and grill for 10 to 15 minutes or to desired doneness, occasionally turning and basting. Serve.

OPTIONS

- Broil 4 inches from heat.

Louisiana Lamb Steaks

NO CARBOHYDRATES   **NUMBER OF SERVINGS: 2 OR 3**

1 tablespoon olive oil
1 tablespoon hot pepper sauce

2 lamb center steaks, cut 1 to 1 ½ inch thick, about ¾ pound each

Cracked black pepper

1. Preheat the grill on high.
2. Combine the olive oil and hot pepper sauce in a small bowl. Brush the mixture on one side of each steak. Sprinkle each steak with ¼ teaspoon of cracked pepper, pressing the pepper in with a spoon.
3. Place the steaks on the grill and reduce the heat to medium. Grill the steaks, prepared side down, for 8 minutes. Brush the uncooked side with the remaining oil mixture, then sprinkle with pepper. Turn and grill for another 8 minutes or to desired doneness. Serve.

Herbed Lamb Kebobs

LOW CARBOHYDRATES   **NUMBER OF SERVINGS: 3**

¼ cup olive oil
¼ cup lemon juice
1 teaspoon basil
1 teaspoon salt
½ teaspoon paprika
½ teaspoon onion powder
½ teaspoon thyme
¼ teaspoon garlic powder

1½ pound boneless lamb, cut into 1 ¼-inch cubes

6 cauliflowerettes (1 cup)
6 1-inch rounds of zucchini (½ cup)
6 small onions
12 large mushrooms

1. Preheat the broiler to high.
2. In a small bowl, combine the oil, lemon juice, basil, salt, paprika, onion powder, thyme, and garlic powder. Pour over the lamb. Cover and refrigerate 6 to 8 hours or overnight, turning occasionally.
3. Alternately thread the lamb and vegetables on six skewers. Broil 3 to 5 inches from the heat for 13 to 16 minutes, brushing frequently with marinade and turning to brown evenly. Serve.

Backyard Lamb Burgers

LOW CARBOHYDRATES   **NUMBER OF SERVINGS: 4**

1 red bell pepper, cored, seeded and cut
into thin strips
½ tablespoon olive oil

1 ripe avocado, thinly sliced
1 tablespoons lemon juice

2 pounds lean ground lamb
¼ cup diced onion
¼ cup minced parsley
1 teaspoon grated lemon peel
Salt and pepper

Sour cream as desired

1. Heat the oil in a small skillet; add red pepper strips and stir-fry until wilted; set aside.
2. Toss the avocado slices in lemon juice; set aside.
3. Preheat the grill on high.
4. Combine the lamb, onion, parsley, lemon peel, salt, and pepper. Form into 4 patties 1-inch thick.
5. Place the patties on the grill. Close the lid and reduce the heat to medium. Grill 7 or 8 minutes per side or to desired doneness.
6. Serve topped with reserved peppers, avocado, and a dollop of sour cream.

Grilled Gyro Burger

TRACE CARBOHYDRATES   **NUMBER OF SERVINGS: 2**

½ teaspoon garlic powder
½ teaspoon pepper
¼ teaspoon onion powder
¼ teaspoon ground cumin
¼ teaspoon salt

1 pound lean ground lamb

1. Preheat the grill.
2. Mix the seasonings and add to the lamb. Mix well then form into 2 patties, about ¾-inch thick.
3. Grill on medium heat for 5 or 6 minutes per side, or to desired doneness.

OPTIONS
- Serve with sour cream and minced green onions.

Roasted Rack of Lamb with Mustard Glaze

NO CARBOHYDRATES   **NUMBER OF SERVINGS: 8**

½ cup Dijon mustard
1 tablespoon soy sauce
1 tablespoon olive oil
2 cloves garlic, minced
1 teaspoon rosemary
¼ teaspoon ground ginger

2 racks of lamb (7 to 8 ribs each)

1. Preheat the oven to 375°.
2. In a small bowl, stir together the mustard, soy sauce, olive oil, garlic, rosemary, and ginger.
3. Trim excess fat from the lamb.
4. Place the lamb, fat side up, on a rack in a shallow roasting pan. Brush on the mustard mixture.
5. Roast for 27 to 30 minutes per pound or to desired doneness and serve.

Grilled Butterflied Leg of Lamb

⅓ **cup olive oil**
⅓ **cup lemon juice**
¼ **cup cooking sherry (optional)**
¼ **cup water**
2 tablespoons finely chopped shallot or green onion
1 tablespoon chopped fresh oregano
1 tablespoon chopped fresh rosemary

6 to 8 pound leg of lamb, boned and butterflied (Have a butcher bone the leg of lamb, then slit the leg lengthwise and spread flat.)

1. Make the marinade in a small bowl by combining the oil, lemon juice, sherry, water, shallot, or onion, oregano, and rosemary.
2. Trim excess fat from the lamb.
3. Place the lamb in a large shallow baking dish; pour the marinade over the lamb. Cover and refrigerate for 8 hours or overnight, turning occasionally.
4. Preheat the grill on high heat.
5. Drain lamb, reserving marinade.
6. Place the lamb on the grill rack directly over the heat. Reduce the heat to medium and close the lid. Turn every 15 minutes and brush with marinade. Cook 40 to 50 minutes, or to desired doneness and serve.

OPTIONS
• Broil the lamb 4 to 5 inches below heat for 35 to 45 minutes, turning every 15 minutes and brushing with the marinade.

Traditional Leg of Lamb

VERY LOW CARBOHYDRATES   **NUMBER OF SERVINGS: 8 TO 10**

5- to 6-pound leg of lamb
3 to 4 cloves garlic
1 teaspoon lemon pepper seasoning
1 can beef broth
1 large onion, peeled and quartered

1. Preheat the oven to 350°.
2. Make small slits in the leg of lamb. Cut the garlic cloves into slices and tuck into the slits. Rub the leg generously with the lemon-pepper seasoning.
3. Place the lamb in a roasting pan. Pour the beef broth and water into the roaster and add the onions.
4. Bake for 25 to 30 minutes per pound, or to desired doneness.
5. Remove from the oven and serve.

Eastertime Leg of Lamb

VERY LOW CARBOHYDRATES   **NUMBER OF SERVINGS: 8 TO 10 SERVINGS**

6 to 9 pound leg of lamb, bone-in
2 cloves garlic, slivered
½ cup lemon juice
2 teaspoons fresh chopped basil
2 teaspoons fresh chopped rosemary OR
*   fresh summer savory*
Salt and pepper to taste

1. Preheat the oven to 325°.
2. Place lamb in a shallow roasting pan. Cut slits in the surface and insert the garlic slivers into the slits. Rub lemon juice over lamb surface. Sprinkle with herbs, salt and pepper; rub into surface.
3. Place the lamb in oven and roast for 20 minutes per pound, or to desired doneness.
4. Remove from oven and serve.

Celebration Leg of Lamb

VERY LOW CARBOHYDRATES   **NUMBER OF SERVINGS: 8 - 10**

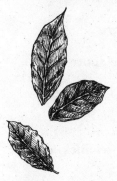

1 clove garlic, crushed
1 teaspoon pepper
½ teaspoon ginger
1 whole bay leaf, crushed
½ teaspoon thyme
½ teaspoon sage
½ teaspoon marjoram
1 tablespoon soy sauce
1 tablespoon olive oil

6-to 9-pound leg of lamb, bone-in

1. Preheat the oven to 325°.
2. In a small bowl, mix together all of the ingredients except the lamb.
3. Place the lamb on a rack in a roasting pan. With a sharp knife, make frequent slits in the surface of lamb. Move the knife from side to side to enlarge the cuts. Rub the herb mixture into each slit. Rub any remaining mixture over the roast.
4. Roast for 20 to 25 minutes per pound, or to desired doneness.
5. Remove from the oven and serve. Pan drippings can be skimmed and served au jus.

Arizona Leg of Lamb

VERY LOW CARBOHYDRATES   **NUMBER OF SERVINGS: 12**

1 cup wine vinegar
1 cup olive oil
2 cloves garlic, whole
1 bay leaf, crumbled
2 teaspoons salt
1 teaspoon rosemary
1 teaspoon sage
½ teaspoon crushed pepper
5- to 7-pound boned, rolled, and tied leg of lamb

1. Combine the vinegar, oil, and seasonings; pour over the lamb. Cover and refrigerate for 12 to 24 hours.
2. Preheat the oven to 325°.
3. Remove the lamb. Strain the marinade and reserve.
4. Place the lamb on a roasting rack. Pour ¼ cup of marinade over the lamb.
5. Roast for about 25 minutes per pound, or to desired doneness. Baste with ¼ cup of the marinade every 20 to 30 minutes. Serve.

Spicy Dijon Lamb Chops

VERY LOW CARBOHYDRATES   NUMBER OF SERVINGS: 4

2 tablespoons olive oil
2½ tablespoons Dijon mustard
2 tablespoons lemon juice
1 tablespoon Worcestershire sauce
1 tablespoon minced garlic
1½ teaspoons liquid hot pepper sauce
½ teaspoon paprika
Salt, as desired

4 lamb shoulder chops, 1-inch thick, about
½ pound each

1. Combine all of the ingredients except the lamb in a bowl.
2. Pour the marinade over the lamb, turning to coat well. Cover and refrigerate 6 to 8 hours, turning occasionally.
3. Preheat the grill on high heat.
4. Remove the lamb from the marinade; place on the grill. Close the lid and reduce the heat to medium. Grill 5 to 6 minutes per side or to desired doneness, turning occasionally and brushing with the marinade. Serve.

Curried Lamb Chops

VERY LOW CARBOHYDRATES   NUMBER OF SERVINGS: 8

⅓ cup lemon juice
¼ cup finely chopped onion
1 tablespoon olive oil
½ teaspoon curry powder
½ teaspoon lemon pepper
¼ teaspoon cumin
¼ teaspoon cardamom
¼ teaspoon ginger
8 lamb loin chops, trimmed and cut 1-inch
thick

1. In a small bowl, combine all of the ingredients except the lamb chops and set aside.
2. Place the chops in a non-metal container or sealable plastic bag and add the marinade.
3. Cover or seal. Refrigerate for 6 to 24 hours.

4. Preheat the grill.
5. Remove the meat from the marinade; place on the grill. Reduce the heat to medium and grill for 5 to 6 minutes on each side, or to desired doneness.

OPTION

• Broil 4 inches under heat.

Pepper-Basil Spicy Lamb Chops

LOW CARBOHYDRATES   **NUMBER OF SERVINGS: 4**

2 teaspoons lemon pepper
2 teaspoons garlic powder
2 teaspoons rosemary, crushed
4 lamb shoulder chops, cut ¾-inch thick

1½ tablespoons olive oil

2½ tablespoons olive oil
1 cup julienne-cut red pepper
1 tablespoon finely chopped garlic
½ cup chopped onion
¼ cup toasted almonds
¼ cup fresh basil, chopped
1 tablespoon red wine vinegar
½ teaspoon seasoned salt
½ teaspoon seasoned pepper

1. Season the lamb chops with the lemon pepper, garlic powder, and rosemary.
2. In a large skillet, heat 1½ tablespoons oil and saute the chops, browning well on each side. Cooking to desired doneness.
3. Remove the chops from the skillet. Cover and keep warm.
4. Wipe the skillet with a clean paper towel, then heat the 2½ tablespoons oil. Add the red pepper, onion, and garlic. Stir-fry for 3 to 4 minutes.
5. Add the almonds, basil, vinegar, salt, and pepper and stir-fry an additional 2 to 3 minutes.
6. Pour over the chops and serve.

Simple Spicy Lamb Roast

VERY LOW CARBOHYDRATES   **NUMBER OF SERVINGS: 4 TO 6**

1 tablespoon olive oil
⅓ cup apple juice
1 teaspoon oregano
⅛ teaspoon ginger
2 tablespoons soy sauce
⅛ teaspoon red pepper flakes, crushed
1 clove garlic, minced
½ leg of lamb, ½ sirloin or full shank (about
   2 to 3 pounds)

1. Preheat oven to 350°.
2. Combine the oil, apple juice, oregano, ginger, soy sauce, red pepper flakes, and garlic.
3. Place the lamb on the rack in a roasting pan. Brush generously with marinade.
4. Roast for 25 to 30 minutes, or to desired doneness. Brush with the marinade several times while roasting.
5. Slice and serve.

Cajun Lamb Roast

TRACE OF CARBOHYDRATES   **NUMBER OF SERVINGS: 3 OR 4**

½ teaspoon salt
½ teaspoon cayenne pepper
¼ teaspoon black pepper
¼ teaspoon chili powder
¼ teaspoon paprika
⅛ teaspoon garlic powder

2 pound boneless lamb roast, sirloin or top
   round

1 tablespoon oil

1. Mix together the salt, peppers, chili powder, paprika, and garlic powder. Rub into the lamb and let stand for 15 minutes.
2. Preheat oven to 350°.
3. Heat the oil to medium-hot and brown the lamb on all sides.
4. Place the lamb in a shallow roasting pan and roast for 35 to 40 minutes, or to desired doneness.
5. Slice and serve.

Curry Lamb Stew

2 tablespoons olive oil
1½ pounds lean lamb meat, cubed

8 ounces fresh mushrooms, sliced
1 medium onion, chopped
½ teaspoon dry sage
½ teaspoon ginger powder
¼ teaspoon salt
⅛ teaspoon black pepper

2 cups canned OR homemade beef broth

1 green pepper, cut into bite-sized chunks
2 medium tomatoes, cut into chunks

½ cup sour cream

1. Pour the oil in a sauce pan and add the lamb; cook together until the lamb is browned.
2. Stir in the mushrooms, onion, sage, ginger, salt, and pepper. Cook together, stirring often, until the mushrooms are soft and the onions are transparent.
3. Add the broth and simmer, covered, 10 to 30 minutes, or longer if you have the time.
4. Add the green pepper and tomato and cook another 5 minutes.
5. Put the sour cream in a bowl. Add the hot mixture, a spoonful at a time, stirring together, until you have about one cup. Then pour sour cream mixture into the lamb. Stir to combine; heat through but do not boil.
6. Serve in bowls.

Even people who do not like lamb love this dish!

Chapter 4

CHICKEN

As a boy, my husband was responsible for chicken chores as his family had 8,000 layers—quite a large flock for the time. The eggs had to be hand-collected daily, cleaned, sorted, and packed in cases for market. Buckets of feed and water had to be hauled, and the chicken houses cleaned. All in all, this was a big job in the days before automation!

Chickens used to provide farm wives with their weekly grocery money, hogs and cattle paid the monthly mortgage bills, and the crop land fed the livestock and supported the farm family. All of this has changed now. Today, few farmers have chickens because corporations have taken over the business. Huge confinement buildings house hundreds of thousands of chickens, with each bird in its own small cage, never able to exercise in the sun.

Fortunately, we have a neighbor who still raises a few hundred chickens the old-fashioned way—they are free-range; that is, they can run around outdoors if they want. This makes his chickens taste very different from the caged factory chicken. Our neighbor's chickens are large, in the 5- to 7-pound range, with huge breasts and wonderfully plump legs and thighs. I usually buy 60 at a time to put in my freezers. Thanks, Terry!

SAFETY TIPS FOR CHICKEN

Poultry should be cooked to an internal temperature of 180°. Poultry is done when the meat is no longer pink and the juices are clear. Thorough cooking prevents the possibility of bacteria growth. (For more information about using meat thermometers, see p. xviii.)

• Frozen chicken should be thawed in the refrigerator. Allow about 12 hours per two pounds of frozen chicken. A 6-pound bird will take about 36 hours to thaw.

• When thawing in the refrigerator, always place the chicken on a plate or a pan so juices do not contaminate other food. Raw juices often contain bacteria.

CHICKEN STORAGE TIMES

	Refrigerated at 40°F	Frozen at 0°F or colder
Chicken, whole	1 to 2 days	1 year
Chicken, pieces	1 to 2 days	9 months
Leftover fried chicken	3 to 4 days	4 months
Leftover pieces, covered with broth	1 to 2 days	6 months
Leftover pieces, plain	3 to 4 days	4 months
Leftover poultry dishes	3 to 4 days	6 months

(Information courtesy of the Iowa State University Extension.)

Basic Grilled Chicken Pieces

NO CARBOHYDRATES   **NUMBER OF SERVINGS: 4**

1 large chicken, cut into serving pieces

1. Preheat the grill on high.
2. Place the chicken pieces on the grill. Close the lid and reduce the heat to medium. Cook until done—when the meat near the bone and the juices no longer look pink—perhaps 45 minutes for a large chicken. Turn the pieces occasionally and move the thinner pieces, like the wings, to a cooler area on the grill or remove when done and keep warm.

OPTIONS

• . If you choose to skin the chicken before grilling, it's best to rub the meat with olive oil to prevent it from drying out.
• Sprinkle pieces with salt and pepper, if you wish.

Lemon-Cumin Grilled Chicken

LOW CARBOHYDRATES   **NUMBER OF SERVINGS: 4 OR 5**

1 large chicken, or 2 smaller chickens, cut up, with the skin
Juice from 3 or 4 lemons

2 to 3 tablespoons olive oil

2 tablespoons cumin
1 tablespoon black pepper
1 tablespoon celery salt
¼ teaspoon red pepper

1. Pour the lemon juice over the chicken. Cover and refrigerate a few hours or all day.
2. Rub the olive oil all over the chicken pieces.
3. Mix the cumin, black pepper, celery salt, and red pepper together. Sprinkle over the oil on all pieces, not too heavily if you prefer a milder spice flavor.
4. Heat the grill on high. Place the chicken on the grill, close the lid, and turn the heat down to medium or low. Cook until done, turning the pieces halfway through. As the smaller pieces get done, move them to a cooler spot on the grill or remove to a warming pan. Serve.

This tastes a lot like rotisserie barbecued chicken—without all the mess!

Grilled Barbecued Chicken

VERY LOW CARBOHYDRATES **NUMBER OF SERVINGS: 4**

> *2 tablespoons butter*
> *½ cup Westbrae Unsweetened Un-Ketchup*
> *2 teaspoons vinegar*
> *1 teaspoon onion powder*
> *1 teaspoon Worcestershire sauce*
> *½ teaspoon gingerroot, minced*
> *½ teaspoon prepared mustard*
> *¼ teaspoon grated lemon zest*
> *1 clove garlic, minced*
> *Dash of Tabasco sauce (we prefer the mild version)*
>
> *1 large chicken, cut up, with or without the skin*

1. Melt the butter in a small skillet; add the rest of the ingredients except the chicken. Bring to a boil, reduce the heat and simmer for 5 or 10 minutes while you cut up the chicken.
4. Preheat the grill on high.
5. Place the chicken on the grill and brush with the sauce. Close the lid and reduce the heat to low. Turn the chicken and baste with the sauce. Repeat several times, stopping about 15 minutes before removing from the grill. Discard remaining sauce.
6. Cook until done—about one hour or longer—and serve.

OPTIONS

• If you have a rotisserie in your grill or oven, mount the whole chicken(s) on the spit and baste with the sauce. Cook on low heat till done, basting occasionally.

• OR place 3 tablespoons hickory wood chips in the bottom of Cameron's Stovetop Smoker, top with the drip tray and rack, brush the chicken pieces with the sauce and place on the rack. Slide on the lid, place the Smoker on the largest burner on medium heat, and cook about 25 minutes per pound. Remove the lid and brush the chicken with more sauce, then place in a preheated oven at 425° for 20 minutes.

The chicken needs be grilled slowly, on low, so the sauce doesn't burn.

Lemon-Herb
Grilled Chicken

VERY LOW CARBOHYDRATES   **NUMBER OF SERVINGS: 4**

1 large chicken, cut up, with or without the skin

⅓ cup olive oil
⅓ cup lemon juice
2 teaspoons paprika
2 teaspoons basil
2 teaspoons thyme
1 teaspoon salt
½ teaspoon garlic powder

1. Make a marinade with the olive oil, lemon juice, paprika, basil, thyme, salt, and garlic. Pour over the chicken. Cover and refrigerate 2 hours or overnight, turning chicken once.
2. Preheat grill to high heat.
3. Place chicken on grill, close lid and reduce heat to low. Turn chicken and baste frequently.
4. When done, remove chicken from grill and serve.

Lemon-Garlic
Grilled Chicken

LOW CARBOHYDRATES   **NUMBER OF SERVINGS: 4**

⅔ cups lemon juice
¼ cup olive oil
1½ tablespoons dried onion flakes OR 1 tablespoon dried onion flakes + ¾ teaspoon onion powder
1 teaspoon thyme
1 teaspoon black pepper
2 teaspoons Worcestershire sauce
2 cloves garlic, minced (increase to 3, if you like more garlic flavor)

1 large chicken, cut into serving pieces, with or without skin

1. Combine the lemon juice, olive oil, onion flakes, thyme, black pepper, Worcestershire sauce, and garlic. Pour over the chicken and refrigerate at least 2 hours or overnight.

2. Preheat the grill on high.
3. Place the chicken on the grill and reduce the heat to low. Turn the pieces occasionally, basting with remaining marinade until the last 15 minutes. Discard unused marinade. Cook until the meat is no longer pink inside and serve.

OPTIONS

- Broiling or baking is not an option with this recipe—it's not nearly as good as grilled.

This is our family's very favorite grilled chicken recipe!

Baked Hickory-Bourbon Barbecued Chicken

VERY LOW CARBOHYDRATES   **NUMBER OF SERVINGS: 2 OR 3**

½ cup Westbrae Unsweetened Un-ketchup
1 tablespoon bourbon whiskey
1 tablespoon Dijon mustard
2 teaspoons Worcestershire sauce
½ teaspoon finely chopped fresh gingerroot
¼ teaspoon natural hickory seasoning
    (check the spice section of grocery store)

3 to 4 pounds chicken pieces, skin on or off
(it works well either way)

1. Make a thick sauce by blending together the Un-ketchup, bourbon, mustard, Worcestershire sauce, gingerroot, and hickory seasoning. Brush over all the chicken pieces.
2. If you have time, marinate the chicken for several hours in the refrigerator. Otherwise, you can cook it immediately.
3. Preheat the oven to 350° or a convection oven to 325°.
4. Place the chicken pieces on a rack in a baking pan; if you don't have the rack, just coat the baking pan with vegetable oil spray and lay the pieces on the pan.
5. Bake, uncovered, for 1½ hours or convection bake for about 70 minutes. Serve.

Easy Baked Parmesan Chicken

TRACE OF CARBOHYDRATES   NUMBER OF SERVINGS: 4

1 ½ cups grated Parmesan cheese
1 teaspoon salt
¼ teaspoon pepper

½ cup melted butter
1 large chicken, cut into serving pieces with
    or without skin

1. Preheat the oven to 350° OR a convection oven to 325°.
2. Combine the Parmesan cheese, salt, and pepper. Place in a small pie pan.
3. Dip the chicken pieces in the butter, then coat with the Parmesan cheese mixture. Place on a rack in a roasting pan. Pour any remaining butter over all.
4. Bake 1½ hours OR convection bake 1¼ hours, or until the chicken is done. Serve.

Baked Parmesan Cream Chicken

LOW CARBOHYDRATES   NUMBER OF SERVINGS: 2 OR 3 SERVINGS

3 tablespoons butter
3 pound chicken parts, skin on

¼ cup grated Parmesan cheese
1 cup heavy whipping cream
½ cup shredded Swiss cheese
Another ¼ cup grated Parmesan cheese
¼ cup grated pork rinds

1. Preheat the oven to 350° or a convection oven to 325°.
2. Melt the butter in a skillet. Add the chicken pieces and cook about 10 minutes on medium, turning until brown on all sides.
3. Sprinkle the grated Parmesan cheese in the bottom of a casserole dish large enough for the chicken to be in a single layer and not touching. Place the chicken in the casserole.
4. Pour off the excess grease from the skillet used to fry the chicken; but do not scrape the pan.
5. Add the cream to the skillet and simmer until thickened, about 10 minutes.

6. Remove the skillet from the heat and add the shredded Swiss cheese. Stir until melted. Pour over the chicken pieces.
7. Sprinkle the remaining ¼ cup Parmesan cheese over the chicken. Top with the grated pork rinds.
8. Bake, uncovered, for 45 minutes or convection bake, uncovered, for 35 minutes. Watch closely the last 5 to 10 minutes to avoid burning. Serve.

Southern Style "Shake and Bake" Chicken

VERY LOW CARBOHYDRATES   **NUMBER OF SERVINGS: 4**

1 cup ground pork rinds
1 teaspoon paprika
½ teaspoon garlic powder
¼ teaspoon ground thyme
¼ teaspoon ground red pepper
Salt and pepper as desired

1 large chicken, OR 2 smaller chickens, cut in pieces, OR 6 chicken breasts

¼ cup buttermilk

1. Preheat the oven to 350° or a convection oven to 325°.
2. Mix together the pork rinds, paprika, garlic powder, thyme, red pepper, salt, and pepper. Place in a plastic bag.
3. Brush the buttermilk on each piece of the chicken and place the chicken in the crumb mixture in the plastic bag. Shake to coat. Place the coated pieces on a broiler pan coated with vegetable oil spray. Do not cover the chicken.
4. Bake for 60 to 70 minutes or convection bake for 55 to 60 minutes, or until done.

Oven "Fried" Chicken
with 4 Variations

TRACE OR NO CARBOHYDRATES

NUMBER OF SERVINGS: 4 OR 5

Seasoned Pork Rind Coating (see below)
½ cup melted butter (or olive oil)
1 large chicken, cut up, Or two smaller
chickens—with or without the skin

1. Preheat oven at 350° or a convection oven to 325°.
2. (See below.) Mix together the pork rinds, cheese, parsley, salt, and pepper. Place in a small pie pan.
3. Melt the butter in the microwave for 30 to 40 seconds on high. Pour into another small pie pan.
4. Coat a rack in a baking pan or a foil-lined baking pan with vegetable oil spray. Or use a broiling pan, coated with vegetable oil spray.
5. Dip the chicken pieces in the butter, then in the pork rind mixture, and place the coated pieces on the rack or baking pan.
6. Leave the pan uncovered and bake for 75 to 90 minutes or convection bake for 60 to 75 minutes, or until well-done and serve.

OPTIONS

Seasoned Pork Rinds Variation # 1
        1 cup ground pork rinds
        ⅓ cup grated Parmesan cheese or Romano cheese, or a combination
        1 tablespoon parsley
        ½ to 1 teaspoon salt
        ¼ to ½ teaspoon pepper

Seasoned Pork Rind Coating: Variation #2
• Follow the above recipe, except make the pork rind mixture as follows:
        1 cup ground pork rinds
        1 teaspoon summer savory
        ½ teaspoon salt
        ¼ teaspoon pepper

Seasoned Pork Rind Coating: Variation #3
• Follow Variation #2, but substitute 1 teaspoon garlic powder for the summer savory.

Seasoned Pork Rind Coating: Variation #4
• Follow Variation #2, but substitute 1 teaspoon paprika for the summer savory.

All of these variations make wonderful, crispy chicken that resembles the crispness of deep fat-fried without the greasy mess!

Baked Chicken with Beer and Tomato sauce

NUMBER OF SERVINGS: 4

1 large chicken, cut up, skin on or off
12-ounce can Miller Lite Beer
8-ounce can tomato sauce
½ of a medium onion, chopped
½ of a green pepper, chopped
2 garlic cloves, minced
¼ teaspoon ground black pepper
¼ teaspoon oregano
¼ teaspoon paprika

1. If you leave the skin on, fry the chicken in a little oil in the skillet to brown it first. Otherwise eliminate this step. Preheat the oven to 350° or a convection oven to 325°.
2. Crowd the chicken pieces into a baking pan with high sides.
3. Mix the rest of the ingredients in a bowl; pour over chicken.
4. Bake, uncovered 1½ hours until done, or convection bake 1¼ hours or until done. Serve with the liquid spooned over the chicken.

OPTIONS
- Use any leftover liquid as a wonderful soup base.

Easy "Barbecued" Chicken

VERY LOW CARBOHYDRATES NUMBER OF SERVINGS: 4

1 large chicken, cut up, skin on or off

2 cups no carb cola beverage
8 ounce can tomato sauce
¼ cup vinegar
1 tablespoon dehydrated minced onion
½ teaspoon celery seed
¼ teaspoon dry mustard
⅛ teaspoon cinnamon
⅛ teaspoon ground cloves

1. Preheat the oven at 350°, or a convection oven to 325°. Place the chicken in an 8- by 12-inch casserole dish, with sides over 2 inches high. Combine the rest of the ingredients; pour over the chicken.

Chicken 153

2. Bake, uncovered for 1½ to 2 hours or convection bake 1 to 1½ hours, turning the chicken pieces over halfway. Serve.

This recipe tastes like it uses a sugary barbecue sauce, but it doesn't! I rarely have cola in our house and I have mixed feelings about using it in recipes, even the kind without any sugar, but I had a bottle left over from a New Year's Eve party and so I experimented with this dish. It was wonderful. Be aware, however, of the artificial sugar content of the pop, and perhaps use this recipe only occasionally. I have such doubts about it that this is one of only two recipes in this entire book that calls for artificial sweeteners.

Beer Baked Chicken

TRACE CARBOHYDRATES　　　　　　　　　　　**NUMBER OF SERVINGS: 4**

1 large chicken or two smaller ones, cut into pieces

⅓ cup Miller's Lite Beer
⅓ cup prepared mustard
⅓ cup vinegar
¼ cup olive oil
½ teaspoon salt
½ teaspoon garlic powder
½ teaspoon onion powder
¼ teaspoon paprika
¼ teaspoon black pepper

1. Preheat the oven to 375°, or use convection bake, if you have it.
2. Blend all of the ingredients together except the chicken. (I like to use my Cuisinart Cordless Hand Blender with the blade.)
3. Spray a roaster pan and rack with vegetable coating to make clean-up easier.
4. Dip each piece of chicken in the beer sauce and place on the rack in the pan.
5. Bake, uncovered for 45 minutes to one hour or until done and serve.

If you don't have a roaster pan, place a wire rack in a lasagna pan or even a cake pan.

Baked Vegetable Chicken with Wine Broth

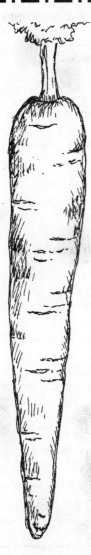

LOW CARBOHYDRATES

**NUMBER
OF SERVINGS: 4**

1 small onion
1 outer rib of celery
½ of one carrot

2 to 3 tablespoons butter
1 large chicken, cut into pieces and skinned
Salt and pepper as desired

½ cup sauterne wine
4-ounce can sliced mushrooms, not drained
2 bay leaves

1. Preheat the oven to 350°.
2. Using the thinnest blade on a Cuisinart, slice the carrot, onion, and celery. Set aside.
3. Melt the butter in a casserole with a lid. (I use a 2½ quart Corningware oval.) Place the skinned chicken in the casserole.
4. Top the chicken with the vegetables; pour in the wine and mushrooms. Place the bay leaves in the liquid along each side of the casserole.
5. Bake, covered, for 1 hour or until done. Remove the bay leaves before serving.

OPTIONS

• Use unskinned chicken pieces if you lightly brown them first in a skillet on the stove with a little butter or olive oil.

• **This entire recipe can be assembled earlier in the day and refrigerated; later, it can simply be popped in the oven.**
• **Save the liquid; it makes a wonderful soup by adding diced celery and cut-up leftover chicken.**

Chicken Baked with Bacon, Wine and Mushrooms

LOW CARBOHYDRATES   **NUMBER OF SERVINGS: 4**

1 large chicken, cut into pieces
6 slices bacon (or more, if needed)
3 tablespoons butter

1 cup red cooking wine
¼ cup water + 1 teaspoon beef bouillon
    granules
1 tablespoon finely minced fresh parsley
¼ teaspoon pepper
⅛ teaspoon paprika
Dash rosemary
8 ounces sliced mushrooms

3 tablespoons melted butter
Additional finely minced fresh parsley for
    garnish.

1. Wrap the bacon around each piece of chicken, securing with a toothpick.
2. Melt the butter in an ovenproof skillet large enough to hold all the chicken pieces snugly in a single layer.
3. Fry the chicken in the skillet, turning to brown all sides. Remove the skillet from the heat.
4. Preheat the oven to bake OR convection bake at 325°.
5. Combine all of the remaining ingredients, except butter in a bowl, stirring well. Pour over the chicken. Drizzle melted butter over all.
6. Place the skillet in the center rack of oven and bake 1½ hours OR convection bake about 1 ¼ hours or until chicken is well done.
7. Serve with mushrooms and a little of the pan drippings, topped with additional minced parsley.

Chicken Baked in Wine Herb Sauce

VERY LOW CARBOHYDRATES   **NUMBER OF SERVINGS: 4**

1 large chicken, cut into serving pieces,
    skinned removed

2 tablespoons butter
2 tablespoons finely diced onion
½ cup white cooking wine

1 tablespoons finely minced fresh parsley
½ teaspoon oregano
½ teaspoon poultry seasoning
⅛ teaspoon tarragon
⅛ teaspoon marjoram

¼ cup grated Parmesan cheese
1 teaspoon paprika

1. Preheat the oven to 350° OR convection bake at 325°.
2. Coat a 13-inch baking dish with vegetable oil spray. Place the chicken in the dish.
3. In a saucepan, melt the butter and add the onion, cooking on medium heat until transparent.
4. Add the wine, parsley, oregano, poultry seasoning, tarragon, and marjoram. Boil 2 minutes or until the sauce is somewhat reduced.
5. Brush herb butter sauce over the chicken; drizzle any remaining sauce on chicken. Sprinkle Parmesan cheese and paprika over all.
6. Bake, uncovered, for ½ hour OR convection bake for 1¼ hours or until done. Serve.

Fried Chicken

VERY LOW CARBOHYDRATES   **NUMBER OF SERVINGS: 4**

1 cup ground pork rinds
1½ teaspoons paprika
1½ teaspoons dry mustard
3 cloves minced garlic
¾ teaspoon nutmeg
½ teaspoon salt (or to taste)
½ teaspoon pepper (or to taste)

1 large chicken, cut up, or two smaller
   chickens, skin cut off
Cooking oil

1. In a small pie plate, mix together the pork rinds, paprika, mustard, garlic, nutmeg, salt, and pepper.
2. Pour one inch of oil into a large skillet and heat to 350°.
3. Dip the chicken pieces in the crumb mixture and place into the skillet. Do not crowd; the chicken pieces should not touch. Fry 10 to 15 minutes, then turn with tongs and fry another 10 to 15 minutes.
4. Remove the pieces to drain on a paper towel and serve.

The inside of this wonderful chicken is moist and tender, while the outside is crispy without being greasy. Delicious!

Fried Curry Chicken

¼ cup ground pork rinds
1½ teaspoons curry powder
1½ teaspoons onion powder
½ teaspoon turmeric
¼ teaspoon ginger powder
¼ teaspoon dry mustard

3 pounds chicken pieces, skin on or off
2 to 3 tablespoons butter or olive oil

½ cup white cooking wine

Sour cream

1. Combine the pork rinds, curry powder, onion powder, turmeric, ginger, and mustard in a small pie plate.
2. Heat the butter or oil in a skillet.
3. Dip the chicken pieces in the spice and pork rind blend and fry in the oil, turning once, until all the sides are browned.
4. Add ½ cup white cooking wine. Cover the skillet and simmer for 30 minutes.
5. Serve each piece of chicken with a dollop of sour cream.

Lemon-Dill Chicken

¼ pound butter (1 stick)
2 tablespoons lemon juice
½ teaspoon lemon zest (optional)
1½ teaspoons dillweed
2 cloves minced garlic
½ teaspoon paprika
⅛ teaspoon pepper
8 ounces sliced fresh mushrooms

1 large chicken, cut up, or 2 smaller ones, skinned or unskinned

1. Melt the butter in a large skillet then add all of the other ingredients except the chicken. Stir and heat until bubbly.

2. Add the chicken pieces. Cover and simmer 30 minutes, or until done.
3. Serve with the sauce and mushrooms on top of the chicken.

OPTIONS
• This would also be good with 3 or 4 pounds of chicken breasts, either bone-in or boneless.

Tomato-Olive Chicken

LOW CARBOHYDRATES   **NUMBER OF SERVINGS: 4 OR 5**

⅓ *cup olive oil or butter*
1 onion, chopped
2 cloves garlic, minced
½ *teaspoon paprika*
¼ *teaspoon pepper*

1 large chicken, cut up, or 3 pounds of
    chicken breasts, bone in or boneless

3 medium tomatoes, quartered
4 ounce jar of pimento-stuffed olives,
    drained and sliced
16 ounces mushrooms, sliced
1½ *cup white cooking wine*

1. Heat the olive oil or butter in a large skillet. Add the onion and garlic, and stir-fry for about 3 minutes. Top with the paprika and pepper and blend.
2. Place the chicken pieces in the pan on medium-high heat. Turn to brown on all sides.
3. Add the remaining ingredients, cover, and simmer 1 hour. Remove the lid for the last 15 minutes. Stir once or twice.
4. Serve with the liquid over the chicken.

Cashew Chicken Curry

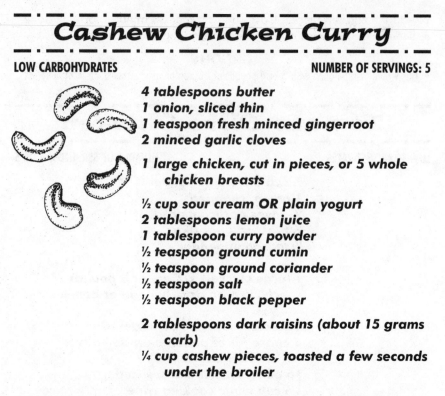

4 tablespoons butter
1 onion, sliced thin
1 teaspoon fresh minced gingerroot
2 minced garlic cloves

1 large chicken, cut in pieces, or 5 whole
    chicken breasts

½ cup sour cream OR plain yogurt
2 tablespoons lemon juice
1 tablespoon curry powder
½ teaspoon ground cumin
½ teaspoon ground coriander
½ teaspoon salt
½ teaspoon black pepper

2 tablespoons dark raisins (about 15 grams
    carb)
¼ cup cashew pieces, toasted a few seconds
    under the broiler

1. Melt the butter in a skillet. Add the onion, gingerroot, and garlic.
   Cook on medium, stirring often, until the onions are softened.
2. Add chicken pieces to the skillet, turning to brown on all sides.
3. In a small bowl, combine the sour cream or yogurt, lemon juice, curry,
   cumin, coriander, salt, and pepper. Pour over the chicken and turn the
   pieces to coat all over. Simmer, covered, on low heat for 45 minutes
   to 1 hour or until done, turning the chicken once or twice.
4. Sprinkle on the raisins and cashews just before serving.

Beer-Tomato Chicken

3 to 4 tablespoons butter
1 large chicken, skinned and cut into pieces
    OR 5 skinned chicken breasts, with or
    without bones

8 to 10 chopped green onions, including
    tops
½ cup chopped celery (about 1 large outer rib)

12-ounce can Miller Lite Beer
14-ounce can tomatoes in tomato juice,
 undrained (check the label for no added
 sugar)
¼ teaspoon thyme
1 bay leaf
Salt and pepper to taste

1. Melt the butter in a large skillet; add the chicken and brown lightly on all sides.
2. Add the remaining ingredients. Cover and simmer for 30 minutes. Remove lid and simmer for 15 to 20 more minutes, until the chicken is done.
3. Remove the bay leaf and serve the chicken pieces in bowls with the delicious broth.

OPTIONS

- After the chicken is browned, slow-cook it in the Crock-Pot on high for half a day or on low all day.

Tangy Skillet Chicken

TRACE OF CARBOHYDRATES　　　　　　　　　　**NUMBER OF SERVINGS: 3**

½ cup vinegar
½ cup no-carb soy sauce
1 clove garlic, minced
Dash black pepper

3 pounds of chicken parts, skinned or
 unskinned

1. Put the vinegar, soy sauce, and garlic in a skillet. Bring just to a boil.
2. Add the chicken, turn down the heat, and simmer about 45 minutes, covered, until the chicken is done. Turn the chicken once, about halfway through cooking. Serve.

Ham & Mushroom Chicken in Wine Sauce

LOW CARBOHYDRATES   **NUMBER OF SERVINGS: 3 OR 4**

4 tablespoons butter
3 or 3½ pounds chicken pieces, skinned

4 ounces sliced fresh mushrooms (about 1½ cups)
½ cup chopped onions
½ cup finely diced ham

¾ cup white cooking wine
¾ cup chicken broth
1 tablespoon dried parsley
1 clove minced garlic
Pepper to taste

½ cup heavy cream

1. Melt the butter in a large skillet. Cook the chicken pieces until lightly browned on all sides.
2. Push the chicken to one side and add the mushrooms, onions, and ham, stirring often until the onions look a little limp.
3. Distribute the chicken pieces evenly over the skillet bottom. Add the wine, broth, parsley, garlic, and pepper. Cover, reduce heat to a medium simmer, and cook 45 minutes or until the chicken is done.
4. Remove the chicken to a serving platter; keep warm.
5. Add the cream to the liquid remaining in the skillet; simmer until thickened. (If no liquid remains in the skillet, add about ¼ cup more chicken broth to loosen the browned bits before adding the cream.)
6. Pour the cream sauce over the chicken when serving.

OPTIONS

• Substitute one drained can of sliced mushrooms in step 3.

Chicken in Lemon Butter

VERY LOW CARBOHYDRATES   **NUMBER OF SERVINGS: 4**

1 stick butter
2 tablespoons lemon juice
½ teaspoon salt
¾ teaspoon paprika
⅛ teaspoon pepper
2 cloves garlic, minced

1 large chicken, cut into serving pieces

1. Combine all of the ingredients except the chicken in a large skillet and mix well.
2. Add the chicken pieces to the skillet and bring to a boil. Reduce the heat, cover and simmer 30 minutes or until the chicken is tender, turning pieces occasionally.
3. Remove the lid and allow the liquid to reduce down to a sauce.
4. Serve the chicken with sauce spooned over.

The sauce is wonderful!

Chicken Cacciatore

LOW CARBOHYDRATES   **NUMBER OF SERVINGS: 4**

½ cup olive oil
½ cup butter
1 large chicken OR two smaller ones OR 6
    pounds of chicken pieces

15 ounce can tomatoes and juice (check the
    label for no added sugar)
1 cup finely chopped onion
1 green pepper, chopped
4 garlic cloves, minced
1 teaspoon salt
1 teaspoon black pepper
½ teaspoon basil

¼ to ½ cup red cooking wine

1. In a stew pot with a wide base, melt the butter with the olive oil.
2. Fry the chicken pieces in the butter and oil for 10 minutes, or until golden brown.

Chicken   **163**

3. Add the tomatoes, onion, green pepper, garlic, salt, pepper, and basil. Bring to a boil, cover and simmer for 45 minutes. Remove the lid and simmer another 15 minutes, or until the liquid is partially reduced.
4. Add the wine and simmer another 5 minutes. Serve.

Easy Chicken in Wine

VERY LOW CARBOHYDRATES   **NUMBER OF SERVINGS: 4**

1 large chicken, cut up
½ teaspoon pepper
½ teaspoon paprika
¼ cup butter or olive oil
1 medium onion, chopped
1 cup white cooking wine
Water

1. Sprinkle the chicken pieces with pepper and paprika.
2. Melt the butter in a skillet. Brown the chicken on one side, add the onions, brown the other side of the chicken and lightly brown the onions, stirring often.
3. Pour the wine over the chicken and add a little water, perhaps ⅓ cup, to have about ¼ inch liquid in the bottom of the skillet. Cover tightly and simmer until the chicken is tender, about 45 minutes. Do not allow the skillet to go dry.
4. Serve with any remaining liquid.

Paprika Chicken

LOW CARBOHYDRATES   **NUMBER OF SERVINGS: 4**

2 or 3 tablespoons butter or olive oil
1 tablespoon Hungarian paprika
½ teaspoon salt
⅛ teaspoon pepper
1 large chicken, cut into pieces, skinned or
    unskinned

1 onion, thinly sliced
¼ teaspoon cayenne pepper

½ cup cooking wine
½ cup heavy cream

1. Melt the butter in a large skillet.
2. Combine the paprika, salt, and pepper and sprinkle all over the chicken pieces. Fry the chicken in the skillet. When one side is browned, turn the chicken and add the onion slices.
3. Pour the wine over the chicken, and deglaze the pan, loosening the bits of browned chicken. Cover tightly and simmer on low for 45 minutes. Uncover and continue cooking for 15 minutes.
4. Add the cream and simmer another 15 minutes, uncovered.
5. Serve with the sauce spooned over the chicken.

Coq Au Vin

LOW CARBOHYDRATES   **NUMBER OF SERVINGS: 4**

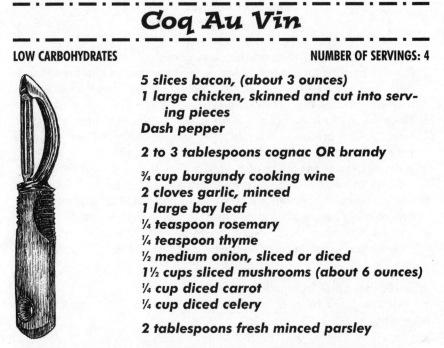

5 slices bacon, (about 3 ounces)
1 large chicken, skinned and cut into serving pieces
Dash pepper

2 to 3 tablespoons cognac OR brandy

¾ cup burgundy cooking wine
2 cloves garlic, minced
1 large bay leaf
¼ teaspoon rosemary
¼ teaspoon thyme
½ medium onion, sliced or diced
1½ cups sliced mushrooms (about 6 ounces)
¼ cup diced carrot
¼ cup diced celery

2 tablespoons fresh minced parsley

1. Fry the bacon in a large skillet until crisp. Remove to paper towels. Pour the excess fat out of the skillet, but do not scrape.
2. Place the chicken in the skillet and sprinkle with the pepper. Fry the chicken on medium heat, turning to brown both sides.
3. Heat the cognac or the brandy in a Pyrex measuring cup in the microwave. Pour over the chicken and immediately ignite.
4. After the flames die down, pour the burgundy over the chicken. Add the garlic, bay leaf, rosemary, and thyme, stir into the liquid. Top with the onion, mushrooms, carrot, and celery.
5. Simmer for 30 minutes, covering the pan for the last 5 minutes.
6. Remove the bay leaf. Sprinkle crumbled bacon and parsley on the chicken and serve with the vegetables and a little sauce.

OPTIONS
• Leave the chicken unskinned.

Chicken   **165**

Super Easy Breasts with Canadian Bacon & Mozzarella

NO CARBOHYDRATES   **NUMBER OF SERVINGS: AS REQUIRED**

Butter
Boneless, skinless chicken breast halves
Canadian bacon
Mozzarella cheese slices

1. Preheat the broiler OR convection broiler on high.
2. In an ovensafe pan just a little larger than the breasts laid single thickness, add 1 tablespoon butter per 2 breast halves, melt the butter under the broiler for a few seconds.
3. Place the raw chicken breasts in the butter, then turn to coat both sides. Lay the breasts in a single layer, snug together but not touching. Put the pan under the broiler.
4. When the top of the breasts are light brown, turn and broil the other side. Be certain the chicken is done and there is no pink left inside.
5. Top each breast half with a slice of Canadian bacon. Place under the broiler a few seconds to lightly brown the Canadian bacon.
6. Turn the Canadian bacon and top with one or two slices of mozzarella cheese. Broil a few seconds to melt the cheese. Serve.

OPTIONS
• Substitute well-crisped bacon for the Canadian bacon.
• Spread 1 teaspoon of Westbrae Unsweetened Un-Ketchup on top of the Canadian bacon before adding the cheese.

Pimento Chicken Breasts

LOW CARBOHYDRATES   **NUMBER OF SERVINGS: 2**

1 tablespoon butter
4 boneless, skinless chicken breast halves
(almost 1 pound)
2 teaspoons canned sliced pimento
¼ teaspoon chicken bouillon granules
½ cup heavy whipping cream

1. Melt the butter in a medium skillet. Cook the breasts on medium-low heat until lightly browned on both sides and no longer pink inside.
2. Top each breast half with ½ teaspoon sliced pimento. Stir the chicken

bouillion granules into the cream. Pour the cream beside the breasts without disturbing the pimento. Leave uncovered and bring the cream to a low simmer without stirring, until thickened.
3. Serve the breasts with the cream sauce.

Smoked Chicken Breasts

NO CARBOHYDRATES **NUMBER OF SERVINGS: AS DESIRED**

Up to 3 pounds chicken breast halves, skinless and boneless
1 teaspoon cherry wood chips

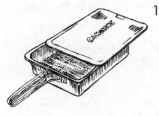

1. Place the wood chips in the bottom of a Camerons Stovetop Smoker. Place the drip tray and rack over the chips. Lay the chicken breasts on the rack. Slide on the lid, leaving it barely cracked open. Place the Smoker on the largest burner on your stove; turn the heat to medium.
2. As soon as the first wisp of smoke escapes from the Smoker, close the lid and begin timing. Cooking takes 20 minutes for 2 breasts; do not overcook.

OPTIONS
• Squeeze fresh lemon juice over the breasts and/or season with herbs or salt and pepper.
• This makes great salad!

This cooking method is fast, easy, and delicious!

Italian Chicken Breasts

VERY LOW CARBOHYDRATES **NUMBER OF SERVINGS: 2**

1 tablespoon butter
2 boneless, skinless chicken breast halves (almost 1 pound)

Philadelphia Cream Cheese
Basil
Garlic powder
Grated Parmesan cheese
Mozzarella cheese slices OR provolone slices OR both

Chicken **167**

1. Melt the butter in a medium skillet. Cook the breasts on medium-low heat until lightly browned on both sides and no longer pink inside. Cool somewhat so that you can comfortably slice the breast nearly in half horizontally to make a pocket for the remaining ingredients.
2. Spread a generous amount of Philadelphia Cream Cheese inside each breast. Sprinkle with basil, garlic powder, and grated Parmesan cheese. Top each with a slice or two of mozzarella cheese.
3. Place under the broiler for a few seconds or until the chicken is heated through and the cheese is melted. Serve hot.

OPTIONS
- Substitute Italian seasoning blend for the basil and garlic.
- Fresh minced parsley would be nice on top of the cream cheese.
- Can sprinkle crumbled bacon on top of the cream cheese layer.
- Top the chicken with pepperoni slices. Then lightly brown them under the broiler before adding the cheese.

This recipe was inspired after eating a similar dish at our favorite restaurant, BozWells, in Storm Lake, Iowa. Thanks, Cindy!

Spinach Chicken

VERY LOW CARBOHYDRATES   **NUMBER OF SERVINGS: 3**

1 to 2 tablespoons butter
2 whole chicken breasts, cut in strips

¼ cup chopped onion
½ teaspoon Worcestershire sauce
¼ teaspoon dried marjoram
¼ teaspoon dried rosemary, crushed
⅛ teaspoon salt (or as desired)
⅛ teaspoon pepper (or as desired)

1 cup chopped fresh spinach

1 tablespoon fresh lemon juice
2 tablespoons finely grated Parmesan cheese

1. Melt the butter in a skillet and add the chicken, stir-fry on medium-high heat until nearly done.
2. Add the onion, Worcestershire sauce, marjoram, rosemary, salt, and pepper. Stir well and cook until the onion is limp.
3. Add the spinach and stir-fry until wilted. Remove from the heat and sprinkle 1 tablespoon fresh lemon over all and stir well. Top with Parmesan cheese and serve.

Artichoke Chicken

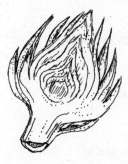

3 tablespoons butter
2 pounds boneless skinned chicken breasts,
cut into 1-inch chunks

1 cup chicken broth
Juice of 2 lemons
2 tablespoons Worcestershire
¼ cup vermouth
2 cloves garlic, minced
1 teaspoon marjoram
1 bay leaf

14 ounce can artichoke hearts, drained and
sliced

1. Melt the butter in a skillet on medium heat. Add the chicken and cook until lightly browned and no longer pink inside.
3. Add the broth, lemon juice, Worcestershire sauce, vermouth, garlic, marjoram, and bay leaf. Cover and simmer for 5 minutes.
4. Remove lid and add the artichokes. Stir-fry until heated through and most of the liquid has evaporated. Remove the bay leaf and serve.

Asparagus Chicken

LOW CARBOHYDRATES   **NUMBER OF SERVINGS: 2**

2 tablespoons butter or oil
2 whole boneless, skinless chicken breasts,
   cut into 1-inch chunks

¼ teaspoon garlic powder
¼ teaspoon dried rosemary, crushed
¼ teaspoon salt
¼ teaspoon paprika

12 spears fresh asparagus, cut into 1-inch lengths
Grated Parmesan cheese
Parsley sprigs (optional)

1. Melt the butter in a large skillet, add the chicken, and stir fry on medium till done.
3. In a cup, mix together the garlic, rosemary, salt, and paprika. Sprinkle over the chicken.
4. Stir in the asparagus and stir fry only till bright green.
5. Place the chicken mixture into a serving dish and top with the grated cheese. Garnish with parsley sprigs, if desired.

This makes a terrific no-fuss meal for entertaining. Just have all the ingredients chopped and ready in advance and stir-fry in front of your guests! Consider serving two entrees—this goes well with Beef Sukiyaki (p. 82).

Easy Chicken Fingers

VERY LOW CARBOHYDRATES   **NUMBER OF SERVINGS: 2**

1½ cups ground pork rinds
¼ cup minced fresh parsley

1 pound chicken breasts, skinless and boneless, cut into 1-inch strips

½ cup Dijon mustard

1. Preheat oven to bake at 425° or to convection bake at 400°.
2. Combine the pork rinds and parsley in a small pie plate.
3. Dip the chicken in the mustard and then into the pork rind mixture. Place each strip on a broiler pan OR in a roaster pan with rack OR on a cookie sheet lined with foil. (Discard any unused pork rind mix.)
4. Bake or convection bake about 30 minutes, or until the meat is done and the coating is lightly browned. Serve.

• To make this a no-carb dish, eliminate the parsley—it still tastes good!

This can be the main course, or you can serve this recipe as appetizers by cutting the strips a little smaller.

Crunchy Chicken
Breast Strips

VERY LOW CARBOHYDRATES   NUMBER OF SERVINGS: 3

1 ½ pounds chicken breasts, skinless and boneless (about 3 halves)

½ cup sour cream
2 tablespoons lemon juice
1 ½ teaspoons celery salt
¼ teaspoon garlic powder
¼ teaspoon onion powder
⅛ teaspoon black pepper
4 teaspoons Worcestershire sauce

2 cups ground pork rinds
1 ½ teaspoons paprika

¼ cup melted butter

1. Preheat the oven or convection oven to 350°.
2. Cut the breasts into 1-inch strips.
3. Combine the sour cream, lemon juice, celery salt, garlic powder, onion powder, black pepper, and Worcestershire sauce in a bowl.
4. Combine the pork rinds and paprika in a small pie plate; mix well.
5. Dip each chicken strip into the sour cream mixture and then into the ground pork rinds. (Discard any unused pork rind mix.) Place each strip on a broiler pan OR in a roaster pan with rack OR on a cookie sheet lined with foil. Drizzle with the melted butter.
6. Bake about 1 hour or convection bake about 45 minutes, watching carefully during the last 5 minutes so it doesn't burn.
7. Remove from the oven and serve.

OPTIONS
• To serve as an appetizer, just cut the strips a little smaller.

Grinding a 6.9-ounce bag of pork rinds in a food processor yields about 4 cups of crumbs.

Tangy Baked
Chicken Breasts

3 tablespoons dehydrated onion flakes
2 tablespoons lemon juice
2 tablespoons melted butter
1 tablespoon vinegar
¼ teaspoon salt
¼ teaspoon pepper
¼ teaspoon thyme
¼ teaspoon garlic powder

1 pound chicken breasts, boneless and
   skinless

1. Preheat the oven to 350°.
2. Combine all of the ingredients except the chicken in a bowl.
3. Place the chicken in a baking dish; pour the lemon and herb mixture over the chicken. Cover with a lid or use foil, sealing the edges.
4. Bake, covered, for 30 minutes, then uncover and bake for 30 minutes more.

OPTIONS
• Instead of leaving the breasts whole, cut them into strips and reduce the baking time a bit.

Marinara Chicken

LOW CARBOHYDRATES   NUMBER OF SERVINGS: 4 OR 5

1 tablespoon butter
2 pounds boneless skinless chicken breasts
¾ cup tomato sauce
½ cup cream
1 to 1½ teaspoons purchased spaghetti
   spice blend
2 cups shredded mozzarella cheese
1 tablespoon Parmesan cheese

1. Preheat oven to 350°.
2. Melt the butter in a skillet. Add the chicken and cook on low, turning
   occasionally. Cook until the chicken is done and the liquid is gone.
3. Place the chicken in an ovenproof casserole dish.

4. Mix together the tomato sauce, cream, and spice blend. Pour half the tomato sauce over the chicken.
5. Top the sauce with the mozzarella cheese, drizzle the remaining tomato sauce over the mozzarella, then sprinkle the Parmesan cheese over the sauce.
6. Bake for 30 minutes and serve.

OPTIONS
- This recipe would work for about 3 pounds of chicken pieces, rather than the breasts.

One whole chicken breast weighs about 6 to 8 ounces.

Tarragon Chicken

VERY LOW CARBOHYDRATES   **NUMBER OF SERVINGS: 4 OR 5**

¼ *cup olive oil*
2 *pounds skinless, boneless chicken breasts*
1 *clove garlic, minced*

½ *cup cooking sherry*
⅓ *cup red wine vinegar*
2 *tablespoons minced fresh parsley*
1 *teaspoon tarragon*
¼ *teaspoon salt*
⅛ *teaspoon pepper*
8 *ounces sliced mushrooms*

1. Pour the olive oil in a large skillet, heat to medium, and add the chicken. Cook for 10 minutes, turning the pieces to brown on all sides.
2. the remaining ingredients. Cover and simmer for 20 minutes and serve.

The tarragon will be quite pungent as it cooks, but never fear—the dish comes out delicately flavored.

Mustard Chicken

VERY LOW CARBOHYDRATES   **NUMBER OF SERVINGS: 2**

2 teaspoons no-carb mayonnaise
1 teaspoon Dijon mustard OR prepared
    mustard
½ teaspoon dried parsley
¼ teaspoon lemon zest
2 large chicken breasts, with skin (about 1
    pound)

2 tablespoons no-carb mayonnaise
2 tablespoons lemon juice
2 tablespoons white cooking wine
1 tablespoon prepared mustard OR Dijon
    mustard

1. Preheat the oven or convection oven to 350°.
2. In a coffeecup, mix together the 2 teaspoons mayonnaise, one teaspoon mustard, parsley, and lemon zest. Gently lift the chicken skin,
   loosening it from the flesh with your fingers without detaching it.
   Spoon half the mustard mixture under each breast skin, spreading it
   over the chicken. Place the chicken skin side down in a baking pan
   just large enough to hold both breasts without overlapping.
3. Using the same coffeecup, mix together the remaining ingredients and
   pour over the chicken.
4. Bake for 30 minutes or convection bake for 20 minutes. Turn the
   chicken breasts skin side up. Bake another 30 minutes or convection
   bake another 20 minutes, or until done. Serve.

OPTIONS
- After you've prepared the chicken for the oven, you can marinate it in the refrigerator a few
  hours—perhaps all day while you're at work. Pop the casserole in the oven, and you have
  a no-hassle dinner while you relax!

Parmesan Sherry Chicken

VERY LOW CARBOHYDRATES   **NUMBER OF SERVINGS: 6**

2 eggs
½ cup heavy cream
1½ cups grated Parmesan cheese
½ cup butter

3 pounds boneless chicken breasts, with or without skin

1 cup cooking sherry

1. Combine the eggs and cream in a bowl.
2. Place the Parmesan cheese in a small pie plate. Melt the butter in a large skillet.
3. Dip the chicken in the cream and then in the cheese. Place in the hot butter in the skillet. Brown on all sides.
4. Add the sherry. Reduce the heat, cover, and simmer for 45 minutes. Serve.

Easy Baked Chicken Parmesan

VERY LOW CARBOHYDRATES   **NUMBER OF SERVINGS: 2**

½ cup ground pork rinds
½ cup grated Parmesan cheese
¼ cup minced fresh parsley

⅓ cup melted butter
1 clove garlic, minced

4 boneless, skinless, chicken breast halves

1. Preheat the oven to 350° OR a convection oven to 325°.
2. Combine the pork rinds, Parmesan cheese, and parsley in a small pie plate.
3. Blend the butter and garlic in a bowl.
4. Dip the chicken first in the butter and then in the pork rind mixture. Place in a single layer on a baking sheet. (Note: Discard any unused pork rind mixture).
5. Bake about 1 hour OR convection bake about 50 minutes until the breasts are tender and lightly browned, and opaque white inside. Serve.

OPTIONS
- I've used this technique with the pieces from one whole chicken, and it's also wonderful. Just be sure to watch carefully that the smaller pieces, like the wings, don't burn.

Chicken Breasts with Canadian Bacon and Red Wine

LOW CARBOHYDRATES NUMBER OF SERVINGS: 3

2 or 3 tablespoons butter
1½ pounds boneless, skinless chicken breast
    halves (about 6)

4 ounces Canadian bacon, diced
1 onion, sliced
¾ cup red cooking wine
1 bay leaf
¼ teaspoon poultry seasoning

2 tablespoons fresh minced parsley

1. Melt the butter in a large skillet and brown the breasts on all sides; push to one side. Add the bacon and onion slices and brown lightly, stirring constantly. Redistribute the chicken in the skillet.
2. Pour in the wine, add the bay leaf, and sprinkle the poultry seasoning over all. Cover tightly and simmer 20 minutes, or until done.
3. Remove the bay leaf. Serve with any remaining liquid; top with parsley.

Chicken Breasts in Cream & Mushrooms

LOW CARBOHYDRATES NUMBER OF SERVINGS: 2

1 to 2 tablespoons butter
2 whole chicken breasts, boneless, and
    skinned (about 1 pound total weight)
Salt and white pepper as desired

⅓ cup chicken broth or water
⅜-inch cube of fresh gingerroot, chopped

1 tablespoon butter
1 cup mushroom slices
½ cup heavy cream

⅓ cup shredded cheddar/Monterey Jack
    blend cheese, or mozzarella or cheese
    of choice
Paprika

Back to Protein

1. Melt the butter in an ovenproof skillet and brown the breasts on both sides on medium low heat. Sprinkle with salt and pepper.
2. Add the chicken broth or water and the gingerroot; cover and simmer on medium heat until the chicken is done and the breast is tender.
3. In a separate, small skillet, melt the additional 1 tablespoon of butter. Add the mushrooms and cook, stirring constantly, for 5 minutes on medium. Add the cream and allow to simmer on low until thickened, without stirring.
4. Preheat the broiler on high.
5. When the chicken is tender, the liquid should be almost gone. If it isn't, simmer the breasts uncovered for a minute or two. Then stir in the mushrooms and cream and simmer, uncovered, for another 2 minutes on low.
6. Sprinkle the shredded cheese over the chicken and pop under the broiler until the cheese is melted and lightly browned.
7. Remove from the broiler, sprinkle with a dash of paprika, and serve.

OPTIONS
• Instead of browning the breasts, omit the butter, add the water or broth, cover, and poach the chicken until done.
• Adding ¼ cup cooking sherry to the mushroom cream sauce before thickening is wonderful!
• If desired, add ⅓ cup chopped onion with the mushrooms.

Do NOT use high heat to brown the breasts; this will toughen the chicken.

Chicken With Pecan Cream Sauce

LOW CARBOHYDRATES   **NUMBER OF SERVINGS: 3**

1 to 2 tablespoons butter
1½ pounds boneless, skinless chicken breasts, cut into 1-inch chunks

1½ cups sliced mushrooms (about 4 ounces)
½ cup diced green onion, including tops (about 2 or 3)
⅛ teaspoon garlic powder
Salt and pepper as desired

½ cup heavy cream

½ cup pecans, whole or chopped, toasted a few seconds under broiler
2 tablespoons grated Parmesan cheese

1. Melt the butter in a skillet and brown the chicken on medium heat.
2. Add the mushrooms, onion, garlic powder, salt, and pepper. Stir until the mushrooms are partly cooked.
3. Stir in the cream and allow to simmer on low until thickened a bit. Remove from the heat.
4. Add the pecans and Parmesan cheese, toss together, and serve.

Saffron Cream Chicken

LOW CARBOHYDRATES   **NUMBER OF SERVINGS: 2**

> 1 tablespoon butter
> 1 pound skinless boneless chicken breasts (2 large)
>
> Dash of thyme, salt, and pepper
>
> ½ cup heavy cream
> 1 tablespoon Westbrae Unsweetened Un-Ketchup
> ½-inch piece of a bay leaf
> ¹⁄₁₆ teaspoon saffron (or less)

1. Melt the butter in a medium skillet and cook the chicken on low until done, turning once or twice.
2. Sprinkle the breasts with a dash of thyme, salt, and pepper.
3. Combine the cream, Un-Ketchup, bay leaf, and saffron. Pour over the chicken and simmer, uncovered, on low for 30 minutes, turning the breasts once or twice.
4. Pick out the bay leaf and discard; serve the chicken with the sauce.

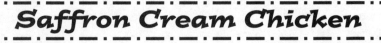
Saffron is expensive, but do remember that you use only a tiny bit.

Chicken Breasts with Lemon Cream Sauce

LOW CARBOHYDRATES   **NUMBER OF SERVINGS: 2**

> 4 skinless boneless chicken breast halves
> Salt and pepper as desired
> 2 tablespoons butter
> 2 tablespoons dry white wine
> 1½ tablespoons lemon juice
> ½ teaspoon grated lemon zest
> ½ cup heavy cream
> 1 cup shredded Swiss cheese OR mozzarella cheese

Back to Protein

1. Set the broiler rack 4 inches below the heat; preheat broiler on high.
2. Sprinkle the chicken with the salt and pepper on both sides. Melt the butter in a skillet; add the chicken and cook until done, browning both sides, all four at a time. Stack the breasts to one side.
3. On low heat, add wine, lemon juice and zest to skillet. Deglaze skillet by scraping up browned bits. Redistribute the chicken to a single layer in skillet, cover and simmer for 5 minutes.
4. Add the cream and simmer on low, uncovered, without stirring, until bubbly and somewhat reduced, about 10 minutes. Occasionally turn the breasts.
5. Top with Swiss cheese and place under the broiler a few seconds until bubbly and the cheese is lightly browned.
6. Serve with the sauce.

OPTIONS

• Serve with lemon wedges, if desired.
• For Chicken Breasts in Lemon Garlic Cream Sauce, add a clove of minced garlic to the wine, lemon juice, and zest before simmering!

Ultra-Easy
Roasted Chicken

NO CARBOHYDRATES   **NUMBER OF SERVINGS: 3 OR 4**

1 large whole chicken, unskinned

1. Preheat the oven to 375° OR a convection oven to 350° OR an outdoor grill on high heat.
2. Place the chicken neck-up on a vertical poultry roaster and set inside a large drip pan for the oven, omit for the grill because it has a built-in drip pan. Bake 15 to 20 minutes per pound OR convection bake 15 minutes per pound Or grill with the lid closed on medium heat. Note: The meat thermometer should read 180°.

OPTIONS

• This technique can be used for a small turkey.
• If you don't have a vertical roaster, spray the rack in a roasting pan with vegetable oil and follow the instructions for baking OR spray the grill rack and lay the chicken directly on the grill.

Roasting a chicken seals in the juices for tender juicy meat with nice crispy skin. A poultry roaster is a vertical cone that holds the chicken upright so it cooks from all sides and inside out. The bird stays moist and it cooks faster. You can use it in the oven or on the grill. At 375°, it takes about 15 to 20 minutes per pound, but be sure to check the internal temperature with a meat thermometer.

Ultra-Easy Smoked Grilled Chicken or Turkey

NO CARBOHYDRATES   **NUMBER OF SERVINGS: 4**

*One large whole unskinned chicken OR
turkey
Hickory wood chips the size of coins,
enough to fill a pan to 1 inch
2 bunches of fresh herbs of your choice (like
cilantro and parsley; herbs are optional)*

1. Soak the wood chips in water for 30 minutes before use.
2. Heat the outdoor grill on high.
3. Place the wet wood chips on a cake pan or pie tin you don't care about or purchase a disposable tin foil pan. Cover tightly with heavy duty aluminum foil. Puncture the foil 6 to 8 times with the tip of a paring knife, but do not go through the pan. Place the pan in the center of your outdoor grill, which is still on high.
4. When the hickory chips begin to smoke, place fresh herbs directly on top of the foil cover and put the whole chicken or turkey on top of the herbs. Lower the grill lid and turn heat down a little. (On our gas Weber grill, we turn off the center burner and set the outer two burners on medium high.)
5. Continue to cook until done, 45 minutes to an hour, depending on the size of the chicken or the turkey. Check with a meat thermometer.
6. Remove the herbs and serve up the hot bird. Let the hickory chips cool completely before discarding.

OPTIONS

• Although it's not necessary, rub a blend of herbs and oil into the chicken or turkey prior to grilling.
• Although we never have to do this, if your wing tips or drumsticks start to get overdone, cover them with small pieces of aluminum foil.

This is so easy and so wonderful—the bird is succulent and juicy!

Roasted Garlic Chicken

VERY LOW CARBOHYDRATES   **NUMBER OF SERVINGS: 4**

⅓ cup olive oil
6 peeled garlic cloves, or more to taste

1 large whole chicken (or two small ones)
Freshly ground black pepper, to taste

1. Preheat the broiler or convection broiler on high.
2. Put the olive oil and garlic cloves in the bowl of a Cuisinart Hand Blender, with blade; mix thoroughly.
3. Rub the oil and garlic liberally into the skin and all the cavities of the chicken.
4. Sprinkle chicken with freshly ground black pepper.
5. Place the chicken back side up in a large roasting pan, uncovered, and place under the broiler or convection broiler for 3 minutes. Turn the chicken breast side up and broil the other side for 3 minutes.
6. Pour any remaining olive-garlic blend over the chicken. Cover the roasting pan and bake in 350° oven for 45 minutes to 1 hour, or until done. Serve.

OPTIONS

- Instead of baking the chicken, cook in your Crock-Pot on high. First, cut up the chicken and add a little water or broth, for food safety. (See p. 46 for Crock-Pot safety)

The chicken smells garlicky as it bakes, but it doesn't taste too garlicky—actually, it is very mild, delicate, and moist.

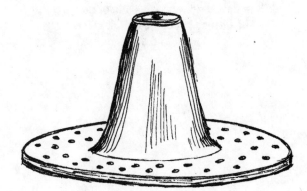

Baked Herb Chicken

⅓ cup butter, melted
1 teaspoon dried thyme
1 teaspoon crushed rosemary
½ teaspoon salt
½ teaspoon pepper
2 tablespoons red wine vinegar
1 tablespoon Worcestershire sauce

1 large whole 6-pound chicken, or two
    smaller ones
One medium onion, quartered

1. Preheat the oven on convection bake, or bake at 350°.
2. Melt the butter in a Pyrex bowl in the microwave for 30 seconds or so.
3. Add the remaining ingredients except the chicken.
4. Using a small food processor or blender, thoroughly mix the ingredients so there are no solids left.
5. Use a baster with a needle to inject the butter mixture under the chicken skin OR loosen the skin and carefully pour the mixture under the skin.
6. Pour any excess butter mixture into the chicken's cavities; stuff the onion quarters in the cavities.
7. Convection bake or bake uncovered about 1 hour or until done, basting occasionally. If the chicken gets too brown, cover it.

> Be sure your herbs are ground well so they to fit into the baster needle without clogging it.
> • The basting sauce makes this chicken very tender and delicious.

Roasted Lemon-Garlic Chicken

VERY LOW CARBOHYDRATES NUMBER OF SERVINGS: 4

1 large whole chicken, unskinned

¼ cup melted butter
3 tablespoons lemon juice
½ teaspoon lemon zest
1 garlic clove, minced
¼ teaspoon salt

1. Preheat the oven to 375° OR the convection oven to 350° OR outdoor grill on high.
2. Place the chicken neck-up on a vertical poultry roaster. Set inside a large drip pan for oven cooking, omit for the grill because of the built-in drip pan.
3. Combine the butter, lemon juice, zest, garlic, and salt. Combine with a hand blender or small food processor with blade. Brush onto the chicken before cooking and frequently as it cooks.
4. Bake for 15 to 20 minutes per pound OR convection bake for 15 minutes per pound Or grill with the lid closed on medium heat.
5. Cook until done. (The meat thermometer should read 180°.) Serve.

This is easy!

Baked Lemon-Garlic Chicken

VERY LOW CARBOHYDRATES NUMBER OF SERVINGS: 4

1 large 6-pound chicken, unskinned
1 lemon, quartered
1 medium onion, quartered
2 cloves garlic, peeled

1. Preheat the oven to 400°.
2. Place the chicken in a covered roasting pan that has been coated with vegetable oil spray.
3. Stuff the cavities with the lemon, onion, and garlic.
4. Bake for 1½ hours or until done. Remove the lemon, onion, and garlic and serve.

The chicken makes its own liquid, and the skin turns a crispy golden brown.

Baked Oregano Chicken

VERY LOW CARBOHYDRATES   **NUMBER OF SERVINGS: 4**

Juice from 2 lemons
1 clove garlic, minced
1 teaspoon oregano
½ teaspoon salt
¼ teaspoon pepper

1 large whole chicken
¼ cup melted butter
½ to 1 cup water

1. Preheat the oven to 350°.
2. Combine the lemon juice, garlic, oregano, salt, and pepper. Rub all over the chicken, inside and out.
3. Place in a covered roasting pan breast side up. Drizzle the chicken with melted butter. Pour the water in the bottom of the pan. Cover and bake for 1 hour, or until done. Serve.

Chicken Simmered in Broth

NO CARBOHYDRATES   **NUMBER OF SERVINGS: VARIABLE**

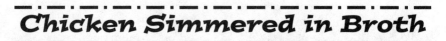

One or more whole chicken(s). I use one or two of our 5- to 6-pound chickens.
Water
1 bay leaf and 1 whole garlic clove per chicken (optional)
Salt and pepper, if desired.

1. Place the chicken(s) in a large kettle with a lid.
2. Add 2 inches of water to the kettle. Add the other ingredients, if desired.
3. Bring the water to a boil, then coven and reduce the heat to a low simmer. Cook until the chicken is done. (I like to cook it about half a day, until the meat is nearly falling off the bones.)
4. To serve, remove the chicken from the water and cut into individual portions.

OPTIONS
- Skin the cooked chicken and sprinkle shredded cheddar cheese on the hot pieces. Salt and pepper to taste—delicious and very easy!

This leftover chicken is terrific for many recipes. Just remove the skin and separate the meat from the bones. (At this point I give the leftovers to our dog and many cats!) Refrigerate the meat in a covered container. NOTE: One of my large 6 pound chickens yields about 6 cups diced meat.

Be sure to strain and save the liquid the chicken was simmered in. Store it in the refrigerator, or freeze in tightly covered containers. It makes wonderful soups and casseroles and can be added to many other recipes. Once cold, the chicken fat rises to the top of the broth for easy removal.

No-Work Baked Chicken

NO CARBOHYDRATES   **NUMBER OF SERVINGS: VARIABLE**

Whole unskinned chicken(s)

1. Put the chicken in a covered roasting pan that has been coated with olive oil.
2. Bake at 350° until done.

OPTIONS

- Use a vertical poultry roaster on a cake pan or jelly roll sheet to catch the drips. Bake as above.
- The whole chicken can be grilled outside on low heat.

Cut off some of the meat and serve hot from the oven or grill. Cool the chicken and separate the meat from the skin and bones. Use the meat for the many recipes that follow.

"BLT" Chicken Salad

VERY LOW CARBOHYDRATES   **NUMBER OF SERVINGS: 2**

6 strips bacon (I use thick cut, hickory-smoked), cooked, drained, and crumbled
2 cups cubed cooked chicken
¾ cup chopped tomato (1 small)
½ cup no-carb mayonnaise
1 tablespoon finely chopped onion
1 tablespoon lemon juice
½ teaspoon to 1 teaspoon purchased barbecue spice blend, optional (I use Cookies' Flavor Enhancer)

Lettuce, as desired

1. Combine all of the ingredients; mix well.

2. Serve over a single lettuce leaf or on a lettuce bed.

OPTIONS

- For more protein, add 2 sliced hard-boiled eggs.
- To fit more bacon in the skillet, cut the strips into thirds.

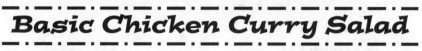

This is so delicious—and you don't even miss the bread!

Basic Chicken Curry Salad

VERY LOW CARBOHYDRATES   **NUMBER OF SERVINGS: 2**

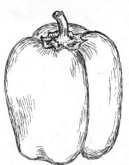

2 cups diced cooked chicken, skinned and deboned
4 green chopped onions plus tops OR 3 tablespoons finely diced onion
⅓ cup no-carb mayonnaise, (Hellman's Original), OR low-carb sour cream
¼ cup diced red sweet peppers
1 teaspoon curry powder

Lettuce or greens, as desired

1. Assemble all of the ingredients except the lettuce in a medium bowl; mix well.
2. Lay the lettuce leaf or torn greens on individual serving plates or in salad bowls. Top with a serving of chicken, neatly mounded.
3. Garnish, if desired.

OPTIONS

- Substitute green bell pepper for the red sweet pepper.
- Add sliced hard-boiled eggs.
- Garnish with a small green onion draped along the side of the dish.

Harvest red sweet peppers or green bell peppers at their peak (or buy them at the market). Wash well, cut out the stems, and quarter. Remove the seeds. Place the quarters in a freezer bag, seal, then place the bag inside yet another and seal it—this keeps the peppers from flavoring other foods in the freezer. When a recipe calls for peppers, remove the number of quarters necessary, rinse in cold water, and cut up as desired. This is very fast and easy—and you'll have peppers available any time you want them!

Chicken Curry Salad
with Black Olives
& Water Chestnuts

VERY LOW CARBOHYDRATES **NUMBER OF SERVINGS: 2**

2 cups diced cooked chicken
½ cup chopped celery (about 2 ribs)
½ cup chopped green onions plus tops, chopped
⅓ cup Hellman's Original mayonnaise OR sour cream
6 or 8 black olives, sliced
1 teaspoon curry powder
1 teaspoon lemon juice
Salt and pepper to taste

Lettuce or other greens

1. Combine all of the ingredients in a medium bowl. Chill.
2. Serve on lettuce leaves or other greens.

Chicken Salad with
Green Olives

VERY LOW CARBOHYDRATES **NUMBER OF SERVINGS: 3 OR 4 SERVINGS**

About 3 cups diced cooked chicken
⅔ cups chopped celery
3 hard-cooked eggs, chopped
¼ cup sliced green olives with pimento
½ cup chopped green onion with tops (or about ¼ cup onion)
1 teaspoon lemon juice
½ teaspoon Italian blend seasoning
¼ teaspoon salt
½ to ⅔ cup Hellman's Original mayonnaise OR sour cream

Lettuce or spinach leaves

Combine all of the ingredients and mix well in a medium bowl. Serve.

- Top the salad with chopped chives or more chopped onion greens and garnish with tomato slices or red pepper strips.
- Top each serving with one teaspoon of sliced almonds.

If possible, make this in advance and refrigerate for several hours to allow the flavors to permeate throughout.

Chicken Curry Salad with Pecans

VERY LOW CARBOHYDRATES   **NUMBER OF SERVINGS: 2**

2 cups diced cooked chicken
⅓ to ½ cup Hellman's Original mayonnaise
1 to 2 tablespoons finely grated onion
1 teaspoon curry powder
Salt and pepper to taste

½ cup pecans (10 grams carb minus 4
    grams of fiber = 6 grams carb)
Lettuce or other greens, (one or more leaves
    per person)

1. In a medium bowl, combine the chicken, mayonnaise, curry, salt, and pepper.
2. In a small ovenproof pan, place the pecans in a single layer. Broil a few seconds.
4. Serve the chicken cold on a lettuce bed. Top with the toasted pecans.

OPTIONS

- Substitute celery seed for the curry powder.
- A little fresh gingerroot paste would be a good addition.
- Add one or two hard-boiled sliced eggs.

Cold Cashew Chicken Salad

LOW CARBOHYDRATES

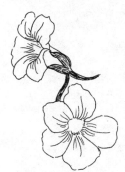

**2 cups diced cooked chicken skinned and
deboned**
½ cup diced celery (about 2 ribs)
**1 bunch diced green onions plus tops (about
6) OR ¼ cup diced onion**
**⅓ to ½ cup Hellman's Original mayonnaise
OR sour cream**
Salt and pepper to taste

Lettuce or greens as desired
⅓ cup cashews, raw if possible

1. Assemble all of the ingredients except the lettuce and nuts in a bowl; mix well.
2. Lay a lettuce leaf or torn greens on individual serving plates or in salad bowls. Top with a serving of chicken, neatly mounded.
3. Place the nuts in a single layer in a small ovenproof pan. Toast under the broiler watching closely so the nuts do not burn. Sprinkle the hot nuts on top of the salads. Garnish, if desired, and serve.

OPTIONS

- Sprinkle paprika on top.
- Garnish with a bright red radish or sweet red pepper strips.
- Substitute pecans, almonds, macadamia nuts, or walnuts for the cashews.

> I like to top each serving of this salad with a single nasturtium blossom from my garden—lovely! When entertaining, I prepare everything in advance and float the blossoms in a little bowl of water until serving time. You can also add a nasturtium leaf or green seed pod—all the parts of the plant are edible and delicious.

Hawaiian Chicken Salad

LOW CARBOHYDRATES   **NUMBER OF SERVINGS: 2**

> **2 cups diced cooked chicken**
> **½ cup diced celery**
> **⅓ cup Hellman's Original mayonnaise OR**
> **sour cream**
> **¼ cup pineapple tidbits packed in its own**
> **juice, drained, OR fresh pineapple**
> **½ teaspoon curry powder**
> **Salt and pepper to taste**
>
> **¼ cup pecans, lightly toasted in broiler**
> **Lettuce leaves**

1. In a medium bowl, combine the chicken, celery, mayonnaise, pineapple, curry powder, salt, and pepper.
2. Neatly mound on lettuce leaves and top with toasted pecans. Serve.

OPTIONS:

• Substitute 1/3 cup chopped apple with peel for the pineapple (about 6 grams carb).

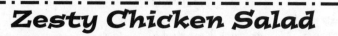
This is attractive served in fresh pineapple shells.

Zesty Chicken Salad

LOW CARBOHYDRATES   **NUMBER OF SERVINGS: 2**

> **2 cups chopped cooked chicken**
> **1 bunch small green onions including tops,**
> **chopped**
> **10 Thompson seedless grapes, sliced**
> **⅓ cup Hellman's Original mayonnaise**
> **¼ cup diced celery, 1 rib**
> **1 teaspoon lemon zest, fresh or frozen**
> **1 teaspoon lemon juice**
> **Dash of black pepper, preferably freshly**
> **ground**
> **Lettuce or greens as desired**
> **Paprika**

1. In a medium bowl, combine all of the ingredients except the lettuce and paprika.
2. Lay the lettuce on individual serving plates, top with neatly mounded chicken mixture, and sprinkle with paprika.

- For the grapes, substitute 1 medium chopped kiwi (9 grams carb) OR ½ of a fresh orange, peeled and with the segments separated and cut into pieces (8 grams) OR ¼ cup pineapple tidbits in natural juice, drained (about 9 grams carb).

Hold back a few pieces of the fruit and some onion tops to garnish this salad. Every time you use a lemon or a lime, be sure to remove the zest first, whether you need it or not. Freeze the zest in a small plastic bag. Later you can remove the amount needed. A great timesaver!

Chicken Vinaigrette

VERY LOW CARBOHYDRATES   **NUMBER OF SERVINGS: 2**

2 cups chopped cooked chicken
¼ of a large green pepper, cut into chunks or strips
¼ of a large red tomato, diced into small chunks
4 to 6 or more mushrooms, cut into thick slices
1 medium green onion plus the tops, chopped

¼ cup olive oil
1 tablespoon lemon juice
1 tablespoon white wine vinegar
¼ teaspoon salt
¼ teaspoon pepper

1 radish, sliced thin (optional)
Lettuce leaves

1. In a medium bowl, combine the chicken, green pepper, tomato, mushrooms, and onion.
2. In a separate small bowl, combine the olive oil, lemon juice, white wine vinegar, salt, and pepper.
3. Pour the dressing over the chicken mixture and combine well.
4. Serve over fresh lettuce leaves. Garnish with radish slices and serve.

OPTIONS

- Substitute a few cherry tomatoes, cut in half, for the tomato.
- Garnish with one or two zucchini or cucumber slices.
- Sprinkle a herb blend of your choice over the salad.

Refrigerating the chicken mixture a few hours before eating allows the flavors to permeate.

Mandarin Orange Chicken Pecan Salad

LOW CARBOHYDRATES   NUMBER OF SERVINGS: 2

2 cups chopped cooked chicken
⅓ cup mandarin oranges in water or juice, drained (11.6 grams carb per ½ cup) OR 1 fresh tangerine, peeled and segmented (about 11 grams carb)
2 chopped green onions, including tops
¼ cup olive oil
4 teaspoons wine vinegar or red wine vinegar (0 carbs)
¼ teaspoon salt, or to taste
¼ teaspoon pepper, or to taste

¼ cup pecans, toasted a few seconds under the broiler (5 grams)
Lettuce or greens

1. Assemble all of the ingredients except the pecans and lettuce in a medium bowl. Mix well.
2. Place the chicken mixture on the lettuce or greens on individual salad plates.
3. Top with toasted pecans and serve.

OPTIONS

• Reserve 1 onion slice and 3 mandarin orange segments per person to place on top of each salad. Arrange them like a flower blossom, with the onion in the center and the orange segments forming the petals. Spread the toasted pecans around the perimeter.

Ginger Chicken Salad with Sesame Seeds

LOW CARBOHYDRATES   NUMBER OF SERVINGS: 2 OR 3

¼ cup Hellman's Original mayonnaise
2 ounces Philadelphia Cream Cheese
1 tablespoon lemon juice (or Real Lemon)
¼ teaspoon dried ground ginger OR ¾ teaspoon grated fresh ginger
⅛ teaspoon black pepper
4 drops Tabasco sauce (we prefer the mild version)

2 cups diced cooked chicken
2 hard-cooked eggs (optional)
¼ cup chopped onion (we love Vidalia)
¼ cup chopped green bell pepper
¼ cup chopped red sweet pepper
4 large black olives, sliced

2 tablespoons sesame seeds, toasted a few
seconds under the broiler

1. In a medium bowl, combine the mayonnaise, Cream Cheese, lemon juice, ginger, pepper, and Tabasco. Blend well.
2. Add the chicken, eggs, onion, and green and red peppers and the olives. Mix together.
3. Serve on a bed of lettuce. Top with toasted sesame seeds and serve.

OPTIONS
• Garnish with fresh parsley and one slice of red pepper.

Chicken Caesar Salad

VERY LOW CARBOHYDRATES   **NUMBER OF SERVINGS: 2**

2 cups diced cooked chicken
2 tablespoons mild olive oil
1½ tablespoon lemon juice
1 teaspoon Worcestershire sauce
1 teaspoon Dijon mustard
1 clove garlic, minced
salt and pepper to taste

¼ cup grated Parmesan cheese
Lettuce

1. Combine all of the ingredients except the Parmesan cheese in a bowl. Toss well.
2. Serve on a bed of lettuce; top with Parmesan cheese.

Lemon Chicken Salad
(hot or cold)

NUMBER OF SERVINGS: 4

1 chicken, cut into serving pieces, OR 6
    breasts, skinned or unskinned
2 tablespoons olive oil
1 tablespoon Worcestershire sauce
1 teaspoon dry mustard
Dash of salt

Lettuce
2 ribs celery, finely diced (about ¼ cup)
6 green onions, chopped, including tops
Shredded cheddar/Monterey Jack cheese
    blend, ⅓ cup per serving, or as desired
Purchased low or no-carb Caesar dressing

1. Marinate the chicken in the olive oil, Worcestershire sauce, mustard, and salt at least 8 hours in the refrigerator in a covered ovenproof pan.
2. Heat the oven to 350°. Place the covered pan of chicken with the marinade in the oven. Bake for 1 hour or until well done.
3. Cool. Separate the meat from the bones and cut into bit-sized chunks.
4. Place the lettuce on a serving plate, top with diced cold chicken, and then the chopped celery, green onion, and shredded cheddar and Monterey Jack cheese blend. Pass the dressing!

OPTIONS
• The chicken is also wonderful cooked on the grill.

> • This is great for people who like lemon but not garlic because, ordinarily, this dish has both.
> • This recipe is quite versatile. You can bake the chicken and serve it hot out of the oven as is for one meal, then cut up the leftovers for a cold chicken salad. Or you can serve whole skinless boneless breasts fresh out of the oven on a lettuce bed topped with the other ingredients for a great hot chicken salad.

Cream of Chicken Soup

NUMBER OF SERVINGS: 4

4 cups chicken broth (can be canned or homemade)
2 cups finely chopped celery
1 clove garlic, minced
Salt and pepper to taste (be careful with the salt if using canned broth)

¾ cup heavy cream
3 cups cubed cooked chicken
½ cup grated Parmesan cheese

1. Put the broth in a saucepan, bring to a boil.
2. Add the celery and garlic, simmer 5 to 10 minutes, until tender. Using the Cuisinart hand blender with blade, process in the saucepan until pureed—this is optional.
3. Add the cream, salt, and pepper; heat just to a boil.
4. Add the chicken and the Parmesan cheese. Stir to blend and heat through without bringing to a boil.
5. Serve in individual bowls. Top each serving with a dollop of stiff whipped cream.

OPTIONS

• Add a 4-ounce can of drained sliced mushrooms with the chicken or use fresh sliced mushrooms sauteed in a little butter.
• Top each serving with a tablespoon of finely grated cheese—we like cheddar.
• Whip cream in the Quick Whip and squeeze out a whipped cream rosette on top of the soup.
• Sprinkle with finely chopped red sweet pepper.

This is a great way to use the broth from the chickens you've simmered for salads and casseroles!

Encore Chicken Egg-Drop Soup

VERY LOW CARBOHYDRATES **NUMBER OF SERVINGS: 3 OR 4**

> **5 cups chicken broth, canned OR home-made + 1 teaspoon chicken bouillon granules**
> **5 green onions, chopped, including tops (reserve a few tops for garnish)**
> **6 mushrooms, finely diced**
> **2 cups diced cooked chicken**
>
> **2 eggs**
> **Dash white pepper**
>
> **2 to 3 teaspoons soy sauce**

1. Bring the broth to a boil. Add the onions and mushrooms and simmer about 3 minutes.
2. Add the chicken and heat through.
3. Crack the eggs into a coffeecup or mug; add a dash of pepper. Beat thoroughly with a fork until frothy.
4. While stirring the soup in a circular motion with one hand, drizzle the egg into the soup in the thinnest stream possible. The egg will look shredded. Let cook on low a minute or two, to set the eggs.
5. Add soy sauce to taste.
6. Serve garnished with reserved chopped onion greens.

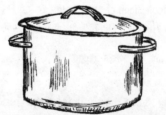

Hot Chicken, Almond and Cheese Casserole

LOW CARBOHYDRATES **NUMBER OF SERVINGS: 4**

> **¾ cup sliced almonds, toasted**
> **4 cups diced cooked chicken**
> **2 cups chopped celery**

2 tablespoons finely minced onion
1 cup Hellman's Original mayonnaise OR
sour cream
1 to 2 cups shredded cheddar cheese

1. Preheat the oven to 350°.
2. Place the almonds on oven-proof pan, spread out. Put in the oven for a short time to toast. Remove and allow to cool.
5. Combine the chicken, celery, onion, mayonnaise and toasted almonds in a bowl.
6. Coat an ovenproof pan with vegetable oil spray.
7. Put the chicken into the pan and bake at 350° for 15 minutes.
8. Top the chicken with the cheddar cheese and return to the oven until the cheese is melted. Serve.

OPTIONS

• Top the cheese with partially crumbled pork rinds and return to the oven for a very short while—be watchful not to burn the pork rinds.

> This dish is great with leftover turkey.

Hot Chicken Enchilada Salad

LOW CARBOHYDRATES   **NUMBER OF SERVINGS: 2 OR 3**

2 cups cubed cooked chicken
¾ cup sour cream (check the label for no
added sugar)
1 to 1½ cups shredded cheddar or longhorn
cheese OR a combination
4 ounce can chopped green chilies, drained
(we prefer mild)
Salt to taste
Lettuce

1. Combine all of the ingredients except the lettuce in a microwave-safe bowl (I use a 4 cup Pyrex measure).
2. Heat on high for 3 minutes, or until hot all the way through.
3. Serve on a lettuce bed.

OPTIONS

• Garnish with a few thin tomato slices.
• Add a 4-ounce can of sliced mushrooms, drained, to the chicken mixture.

> This is extremely quick and easy!

Hot Chicken-Asparagus Salad

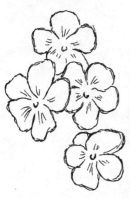

1½ cup fresh asparagus, cut into one inch pieces
2 to 3 cups diced cooked chicken (about ½ of a large chicken); (can be hot from baking or simmering)
⅓ cup slivered almonds
3 green onions, chopped, including tops
Salt and pepper to taste
1½ tablespoons white wine tarragon vinegar OR white wine vinegar
1 tablespoon lemon juice OR Real Lemon
1 teaspoon lemon zest (the amount from 1 lemon; you can use frozen zest)
Lettuce or greens of choice

1. Steam or boil the asparagus until barely cooked and still a bit crisp. Drain.
2. Place the chicken and asparagus in the pan used to cook the asparagus. Cover and place the pan on a burner on the lowest setting to keep the food warm.
3. Toast the almonds a few seconds in the broiler, then add to the chicken and asparagus.
4. Add the rest of the ingredients. Remove the pan from the stove and stir well.
5. Serve on top of lettuce or greens, or a combination.

OPTIONS

• I make this dish in the spring using fresh asparagus, onions, and lettuce from my garden. At the same time of year, the wild violets are in bloom with blossoms that are violet, lavender or white. These are edible and lovely on this salad!
• Garnish each serving with a fresh lemon wedge.

If using a roasted chicken, leave the chicken in the roaster on the counter, covered, while preparing the asparagus and almonds. By waiting a few minutes, the chicken cuts more easily.

Chicken with Caper Cream Sauce

LOW CARBOHYDRATES   **NUMBER OF SERVINGS: 3 OR 4**

1 whole hot chicken, simmered or baked

½ cup white cooking wine
*8 ounces fresh sliced mushrooms or 8
    ounces canned, drained*
⅓ cup finely diced onion
1 clove garlic, minced

1 cup heavy cream
1 tablespoon Dijon mustard
1 tablespoon capers
½ teaspoon dried dill weed
⅛ teaspoon black pepper

1. In a saucepan on medium heat, cook the wine, mushrooms, onion, and garlic together until the liquid is reduced by half.
2. Add the heavy cream, mustard, capers, dill weed, and pepper. Whisk until well-blended.
3. Cook 3 to 5 minutes, until thickened, without stirring.
4. Serve hot chicken meat as desired: with or without the skin, on or off the bones. Pour hot sauce over each serving.

OPTIONS

• Instead of using a whole chicken, substitute about 2 pounds of chicken breasts, simmered in a covered pan in a little water. This is great for guests!

Chicken "Pizza"

2 cups chopped cooked chicken
½ cup sour cream (check the label for no
**   added sugar)**
1 cup mozzarella cheese, shredded
1 clove garlic, minced
¼ teaspoon cumin
⅛ teaspoon Tabasco sauce(we use the mild
**   variety)**

6 or 9 black olives
⅓ cup chopped green onion, including tops
1/2 cup grated Parmesan cheese
¾ to 1 cup additional shredded mozzarella
**   cheese**

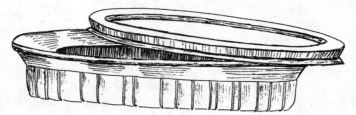

1. Preheat the oven to 450°.
2. In a bowl, mix together the chicken, sour cream, cheese, garlic, cumin, and Tabasco sauce.
3. Spray a vegetable coating on 2 or 3 individual ovenproof serving dishes or porcelain au gratins. Divide the mixture between the serving dishes and spread edge-to-edge, firmly pressing and smoothing the chicken. Heat in the oven for 5 minutes.
4. Remove from the oven and top each "pizza" with 2 or 3 sliced black olives, chopped green onion, then the parmesan,—and finally—the additional mozzarella cheese. Return to the oven for another 5 minutes, or until the cheese melts.
5. Serve on a charger plate or on hot pads, warning people that the dish is hot!

Encore Chicken

VERY LOW CARBOHYDRATES   **NUMBER OF SERVINGS: 1 PER CUP OF CUBED CHICKEN**

*Leftover cooked chicken that had been pre-
pared any way, cubed*
Onion powder or garlic powder to taste
Shredded cheddar cheese
Lettuce (optional)

1. Combine the chicken, onion, or garlic powder and cheese in microwave-
   safe bowl. Cover with waxed paper and heat through in microwave.
2. Serve the warm chicken on a bed of lettuce or as the main protein course.

OPTIONS

- You can substitute almost any preferred shredded cheese in this recipe.

This is super quick!

Encore Smoked Chicken

NO CARBOHYDRATES   **NUMBER OF SERVINGS: VARIABLE**

Leftover cooked chicken
*½ to 1 teaspoon Camerons Hickory or other
finely ground wood chips*

1. Place the wood chips in the bottom of a
   Camerons Stovetop Smoker. Place the drip tray
   and rack over the chips. Lay the chicken on the
   rack. Slide on the lid, leaving it barely cracked
   open. Place the Smoker on the largest burner
   on your stove; turn the heat to medium. (Note:
   Although the smoke will not escape into your
   kitchen, I run my exhaust fan on low while I use my smoker.)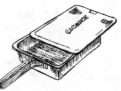
2. Once the first wisp of smoke emerges, close the lid and set the timer
   to 10 minutes.
3. The chicken will be moist and delicately flavored!

OPTIONS

- The smoked chicken can also be cut into strips and served on a lettuce bed with your choice of
  low/no-carb dressings, topped with shredded cheddar and perhaps a little onion. Terrific and fast!

**The day I experimented with this recipe, I didn't have enough chicken for two full
servings, so I added a slab of cured ham to the smoker alongside the chicken—it
was wonderful!**

Encore Chicken a la King

2 tablespoons butter
½ of a green pepper, chopped
1 cup sliced mushrooms
½ cup chicken broth OR ½ cup water + 1
    teaspoon granulated chicken bouillon
2 cups diced cooked chicken
2 tablespoons diced pimento
¼ teaspoon black pepper
½ cup sour cream OR ¼ cup cream + ¼ cup
    sour cream
1 egg yolk
4 teaspoons cooking sherry

1. Melt the butter in a medium skillet; add the green pepper and mushrooms and stir-fry until tender.
2. Add the broth, chicken pimento, and black pepper; bring just to a boil.
3. Combine the sour cream and egg yolk in a small bowl. Spoon a little of the hot sauce into the sour cream and stir; repeat until you double the quantity. Pour the sour cream mixture into the skillet, stir, and heat through but do not boil.
4. Stir in the cooking sherry and serve.

OPTIONS
• Garnish with a sprig of parsley, if desired.

This takes under 20 minutes to make and is really great!

Creamed Chicken and Broccoli

2 tablespoons butter
2 cups broccoli, cut up
4 ounces of mushrooms, sliced
2 cups diced cooked chicken

1 cup heavy whipping cream
¼ cup grated Parmesan cheese
¾ teaspoon Worcestershire sauce
¼ teaspoon nutmeg

¼ cup additional Parmesan cheese

1. Melt the butter in a medium skillet. Add the broccoli and the mushrooms and cook together 2 or 3 minutes, stirring often. Toss in the chicken and stir to heat through.
2. In a small bowl, mix together the cream, 1/4 cup Parmesan cheese, Worcestershire sauce and nutmeg.
3. Add the cream mixture to the skillet with the chicken and broccoli. Mix together, then simmer on low without stirring until somewhat thickened.
4. Serve individual portions and top with the additional Parmesan cheese.

OPTIONS
• If you're in a pinch, substitute canned sliced mushrooms. But be sure to drain them first.

Freshly grated nutmeg is far superior to packaged ground nutmeg, and it's so easy to make if you have a nutmeg grater that is always loaded and ready to use with just a turn of the handle. The grater can also be used to grind other nut meats, such as macadamia, almonds, and pecans.

Baked Chicken Casserole with Celery and Water Chestnuts

LOW CARBOHYDRATES   **NUMBER OF SERVINGS: 3 OR 4**

>   2 cups diced cooked chicken
>   ½ cup sliced water chestnuts (one 4 ounce can)
>   ½ chopped celery
>   2 or 3 hard-cooked eggs, chopped
>   one 2 ounce jar chopped pimento, drained
>   1 cup heavy cream

1. Preheat oven to 350°.
2. Spray a 9-inch, 2-quart casserole with vegetable coating.
3. Mix all of the ingredients together and place in the casserole.
4. Bake for 45 minutes until hot and bubbly, and serve.

OPTIONS
• Top with 1 cup of a shredded cheese blend, if desired.

Creamed Pimento Chicken

LOW CARBOHYDRATES   **NUMBER OF SERVINGS: 3 OR 4**

1 cup heavy cream (½ pint carton)
3 cups cubed cooked chicken (about ½ of a
    large chicken)
2-ounce jar of chopped pimento, not
    drained
salt and pepper to taste

1 to 1½ cups shredded cheddar cheese
one bunch chopped green onions, tops and
    all

1. Place the cream in a skillet and simmer on low without stirring until thickened, about 5 minutes.
2. Add the chicken, pimento, salt, and pepper. Stir together, and cook on low until heated through.
3. Serve topped with shredded cheddar and chopped green onions.

OPTIONS
• Add 1 small can of sliced mushrooms, drained, with the chicken.

Creamed Chicken with Sherry and Mushrooms

LOW CARBOHYDRATES   **NUMBER OF SERVINGS: 2 OR 3 SERVINGS**

1 to 2 tablespoons butter
1½ cups sliced fresh mushrooms
1 cup chicken broth
1 cup heavy cream
2 cups diced cooked chicken
¼ cup cooking sherry
Dash of nutmeg, fresh ground if possible

1. Melt the butter in a skillet.
2. Add the mushrooms and cook on medium heat for about 5 minutes, stirring occasionally.
3. Stir in the chicken broth and reduce by half on medium heat.
4. Add the cream and reduce the heat to a simmer. Cook until the sauce is thickened a bit.
5. Stir in the chicken, sherry, and dash of ground nutmeg. Heat through and serve.

• Substitute a large can of sliced mushrooms, drained, for the fresh mushrooms.

This is a good use for the broth created when you originally cooked your chicken.

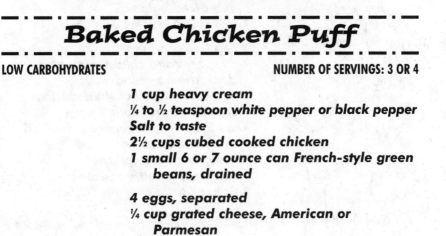

Baked Chicken Puff

LOW CARBOHYDRATES   **NUMBER OF SERVINGS: 3 OR 4**

1 cup heavy cream
¼ to ½ teaspoon white pepper or black pepper
Salt to taste
2½ cups cubed cooked chicken
1 small 6 or 7 ounce can French-style green beans, drained

4 eggs, separated
¼ cup grated cheese, American or Parmesan

1. Preheat oven to 375°.
2. Simmer the cream, pepper and salt until thickened in a medium oven-proof skillet.
3. Add the chicken and green beans to the skillet. Stir together.
4. In a small bowl, whisk together the egg yolks and the grated cheese.
5. Put the whites in another bowl and beat with a mixer until stiff.
6. Fold the egg yolk and cheese mixture into the whites.
7. Pile the egg yolk and egg white mixture over the chicken, spreading it from side to side and smoothing the top.
8. Place the skillet in the oven and bake for 20 minutes. Serve immediately.

OPTIONS
• Add 1 tablespoon minced dried onion OR 2 or 3 chopped whole green onions with tops OR 2 tablespoons finely diced fresh onions to the chicken mixture.
• Add 1 small can of sliced mushrooms, drained, to the chicken mixture.
• Substitute a 14.5-ounce can of green beans for the smaller size (about 14 grams of carbs).
• Sprinkle about ½ cup of shredded cheese on top of the chicken mixture before topping with the egg mixture.

This is rather like having a pastry crust topping, but there is no flour!

Stovetop Chicken Casserole

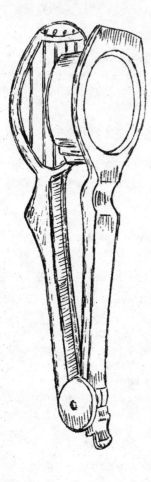

1 tablespoon butter
⅔ cup diced onion
1 cup sliced mushrooms.

1 cup heavy cream
1 cup shredded cheddar/Monterey
  Jack cheese blend
2 to 3 cups cubed cooked chicken
2 chopped hard-boiled eggs
1- to 2-ounce jar pimento, drained
½ teaspoon paprika
¼ teaspoon white pepper
¼ teaspoon poultry seasoning
Salt to taste

1. Melt the butter in a small skillet. Add the onion and cook on medium for 2 to 3 minutes, stirring occasionally. Add the mushrooms and stir-fry another 2 to 3 minutes.
2. Place the cream in a medium skillet and bring to a low simmer without stirring, allowing it to thicken a bit.
3. Add the onions, mushrooms, and remaining ingredients to the cream and stir together. Heat through, but do not boil. Serve.

Fancy Chicken Casserole

VERY LOW CARBOHYDRATES   **NUMBER OF SERVINGS: 2**

⅓ *cup pecans*

2 *cups chopped cooked chicken*
½ *to 1 cup diced celery*
⅓ *to ½ cup Hellman's Original mayonnaise*
    OR sour cream
1 *to 2 tablespoons lemon juice*
½ *teaspoon grated lemon zest*
¼ *teaspoon black pepper*

1 *cup crumbled pork rinds*

1. Set the oven to 375°.
2. Spread the pecans on a small oven-proof pan and bake for 5 minutes.
3. Mix the pecans with the remaining ingredients (except the pork rinds) together and place in a 1½ quart ovenproof casserole.
4. Top with the pork rinds and bake for 15 to 20 minutes, or until hot throughout. Serve.

OPTIONS
• Substitute almonds for the pecans, or eliminate the nuts entirely.
• Other possible additions; include 2 or 3 chopped hard-cooked eggs, pimento, onion, or green onion.
• Sprinkle 1 cup of shredded cheese on top of the chicken mixture before topping with the pork rinds.

I put the pork rinds in my Cuisinart and pulsate the blade a few times until the rinds reach the desired consistency; I usually do an entire bag at one time. Then I store the remainder in a tightly-closed container for future use.

Chicken & Ham with Green Peppers

LOW CARBOHYDRATES   **NUMBER OF SERVINGS: 3 OR 4**

2 *tablespoons butter or olive oil*
1 *green pepper, cut into ½ inch squares*
1 *onion, cut up*
1 *clove garlic, minced*

1½ *cups cubed cured ham, about ½ pound;*
    (check the label for no added sugar)

2 cups cubed cooked chicken
2 cups chicken broth (homemade OR
canned)
1 teaspoon Worcestershire sauce
¼ teaspoon thyme
¼ teaspoon black pepper, freshly ground if
possible
¼ teaspoon Tabasco sauce (we prefer the
mild)

1. Melt the butter in a skillet on medium heat and add the pepper, onion and garlic, stirring frequently.
2. Add the remaining ingredients and cook on medium until the liquid is reduced by half. Serve.

OPTIONS
• If you like spicier food, double the Worcestershire sauce, thyme, black pepper, and Tabasco sauce.

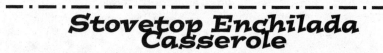

Stovetop Enchilada Casserole

LOW CARBOHYDRATES   **NUMBER OF SERVINGS: 3**

2 cups diced cooked chicken
⅔ cup cream
½ teaspoon chicken bouillon granules
4-ounce can chopped green chilies
½ cup chopped onion

1 cup shredded cheddar cheese

1. Combine all of the ingredients except the cheese in a medium saucepan. Bring to a boil and reduce heat to a low simmer until thickened.
2. Top with the cheese and serve.

OPTIONS
• Garnish with a few thin tomato slices.

This is super fast and tasty!

Chapter 5

TURKEY

We have many friends around our area who raise turkeys—lots of turkeys! So we are well supplied with wonderful turkey meat. We especially like the tenderloins, also called turkey fillets, which are strips of breast meat with no fat, gristle, or skin—wonderful for many recipes!

When buying a turkey, allow 1 pound of meat per person. But why not get a bird large enough for leftovers? You can make a variety of dishes with minimal time and effort. If you can't use all the meat within 3 or 4 days, freeze it.

SAFETY TIPS FOR TURKEY

• Do not thaw a frozen turkey on the counter. It should be thawed in the refrigerator.

• Do not refreeze a frozen turkey that has been thawed unless it has been thoroughly cooked.

• Do not cook a frozen turkey until it has thawed in the refrigerator.

• When thawing in the refrigerator, always place the turkey on a pan so the juices do not contaminate other food. Raw juices often contain bacteria.

MORE TURKEY SAFETY TIPS
from the Iowa Turkey Federation

• Keep the turkey frozen (0° F or lower) or refrigerated (40° F or lower) until cooking or baking.

• Always use a meat thermometer to check the temperature. To be safe to eat, the internal temperature should reach at least 160° F in the deepest part of the breast or 180° F in the thigh. The juices should be clear.

• Never let a raw or cooked turkey stand at room temperature or in a warm oven at less than 200° F or in a holding device at less than 140° F.

• Cooked and cooled turkey products must be reheated to safe temperatures (165° F) before serving or kept cold (40° F or less) if served cold. (The temperature range between 40 and 165° F is where bacteria can grow rapidly.)

• Cut or hold only the amount of turkey that can be served within a 20- to 30-minute period.

• Clean cutting surfaces, knives, pans, cutting equipment, and thermometers frequently; sanitize after each use or between each type of food.

• Keep your hands, face, hair, and personal clothing clean. Wash your hands frequently and thoroughly.

From the Iowa State University Extension

THAWING TIME

For a whole turkey, allow about 24 hours for every 5 pounds.

8 to 12 pounds—1 to 2 days
12 to 16 pounds—2 to 3 days
16 to 20 pounds—3 to 4 days
20 to 24 pounds—4 to 5 days

ROASTING TIME

For a whole turkey, with no bread stuffing, baked at 325°F:

8 to 12 pounds 2¾ to 3 hours
12 to 14 pounds 3 to 3¾ hours
14 to 18 pounds 3¾ to 4¼ hours
18 to 20 pounds 4¼ to 4½ hours
20 to 24 pounds 4½ to 5 hours

Note: These times are approximate and should always be used in conjunction with a properly placed thermometer. For more information about using meat thermometers, see p. xviii.

Basic Grilled Turkey Fillets

NO CARBOHYDRATES   **NUMBER OF SERVINGS: AS DESIRED**

Turkey fillets

Olive oil

1. Preheat grill on high.
2. Brush olive oil on the fillets. Place on the grill and reduce the heat to
   medium. Turn once or twice. The meat is done in 20 to 30 minutes, or
   when the juices run clear and the center is no longer pink.

ALTERNATIVE COOKING METHODS
for all grilled turkey fillet recipes:

• Oven Broiler. It takes about the same amount of total time, although you should turn the fillets often to prevent burning or drying. With a convection broiler, reduce the time by one-fourth.
• Microwave. Use the "brown" setting or the microwave/convection setting, if you have one, according to manufacturer's directions. Turn once or twice while cooking. This is not my favorite method because I feel the microwave changes the texture and flavor of the protein.

OPTIONS
• Serve with prepared mustard, diced onion, or Westbrae Unsweetened Un-Ketchup.

Turkey fillets, also known as turkey tenderloins or turkey breast steaks, are a wonderful all-white meat with no fat, gristle, bone, or skin. They can be used in many ways, and I keep a quantity in my freezer at all times.

Herbed Turkey Fillets

NO CARBOHYDRATES   **NUMBER OF SERVINGS: AS DESIRED**

Turkey fillets
Olive oil
*Dash herb or herb blend of choice: onion
powder, Montreal Chicken Seasoning,
Mesquite Chicken Seasoning, lemon-
pepper, or Rotisserie Chicken Seasoning
(our favorite)*

1. Preheat the grill on high.
2. Brush olive oil on the fillets. Sprinkle with the desired herb or herb
   blend. Place on the grill and reduce the heat to medium-low so the
   herbs do not burn. Done in 25 to 30 minutes, or when the juices run
   clear and the center is no longer pink.

OPTIONS
• Serve with prepared mustard, diced onion, or Westbrae Unsweetened Un-Ketchup.

Barbecued Turkey Fillets

VERY LOW CARBOHYDRATES   **NUMBER OF SERVINGS: 3 OR 4**

> **1 tablespoon purchased Barbecue Spice Blend**
> **½ cup Westbrae Unsweetened Un-Ketchup OR tomato sauce**
> **1 or 1½ pounds turkey fillets**

1. Preheat the grill on high.
2. Combine the Barbecue Spice Blend and Un-Ketchup. Brush on the fillets.
3. Place the fillets on the grill and reduce the heat to low so the sauce does not burn. Cook for about 30 minutes, or until the juices run clear and the center is no longer pink. Serve.

Fourth-of-July Turkey Fillets

TRACE OF CARBOHYDRATES   **NUMBER OF SERVINGS: 3 OR 4**

> **2 tablespoons no-carb soy sauce**
> **2 tablespoons olive oil**
> **2 tablespoons cooking sherry**
> **1 tablespoon lemon juice**
> **1 teaspoon dried minced onion**
> **¼ teaspoon minced ginger OR ⅛ teaspoon powdered ginger**
> **Dash black pepper**
> **1½ pounds turkey fillets**

1. Mix all of the ingredients (except turkey) to make a marinade; stir well.
2. Pour the marinade over turkey, turning to coat all sides. Cover and refrigerate at least 2 hours, (up to 12 hours), or freeze until needed, thawing in the refrigerator.
3. Preheat the grill on high.
4. Place the fillets on the grill and reduce the heat to medium or low. Watch closely to prevent burning or flare-ups. Turn the fillets once or twice. Cook for about 30 minutes, or until the center is no longer pink. Serve.

> This is an all-time favorite. A similar recipe is often used in our hometown for large community gatherings, where church groups set up huge grills in the park and cook hundreds of pounds of turkey fillets for sale during the Fourth of July or other festivities. Wonderful!

Encore Turkey & Cheese

½ tablespoon butter
⅓ to ½ pound cooked turkey
½ cup shredded cheddar OR 3 cheese
        combo, like cheddar, monterey, jack and
        colby
2 slices fried bacon

1. Preheat the broiler.
2. Place the butter in a small ovensafe casserole; place under the broiler for a few seconds until melted.
3. Place the turkey over the butter. Heat a few seconds under the broiler.
4. Top the turkey with cheddar cheese or 3-cheese combo. Return to the broiler until the cheese is melted.
5. Top with the bacon and serve.

OPTIONS

- Substitute Canadian bacon for the bacon. There is no need to fry it first; after the cheese has melted, place the Canadian bacon on top and return the pan to the broiler a few more seconds.

NOTE TO READER
For more ideas on using leftover turkey, see Encore Chicken recipes, starting on p. 185. Cooked turkey and chicken can be interchangeable.

Easy Wine-Italian Turkey Fillets

TRACE OF CARBOHYDRATES   **NUMBER OF SERVINGS: 3 OR 4**

¾ cup low-carb Italian dressing (see p. 296)
¾ cup red cooking wine

1½ pounds turkey fillets

1. Combine the salad dressing and the wine to make a marinade.
2. Pour the marinade over the turkey, turning to coat all sides. Cover and refrigerate at least 2 hours, (up to 12 hours); or freeze until needed, thawing in the refrigerator.
3. Preheat the grill on high.
4. Place the fillets on the grill. Close the lid and reduce the temperature to medium or low. Watch closely to prevent burning or flare-ups. Turn the fillets once or twice. Cook for about 30 minutes or until the center is no longer pink. Serve.

Tomato-Italian Turkey Fillets

VERY LOW CARBOHYDRATES   **NUMBER OF SERVINGS: 2**

2 tablespoons Westbrae Unsweetened Un-
Ketchup OR tomato sauce
Dash dried basil
Dash dried oregano
Dash garlic powder
1 pound Turkey fillets
2 tablespoons grated Romano cheese OR
Parmesan OR mozzarella

1. Preheat the grill on high.
2. Brush Un-Ketchup or the tomato sauce on the fillets. Sprinkle with the basil, oregano, and garlic powder.
3. Place the fillets on the grill and reduce the heat to low so the Un-Ketchup does not burn. Cook for about 40 minutes or until the juices run clear and the center is no longer pink.
4. Remove the fillets from the grill and immediately sprinkle with the shredded cheese. Serve.

Classic French Turkey Fillets

TRACE OF CARBOHYDRATES   NUMBER OF SERVINGS: 3 OR 4

> ½ cup white cooking wine
> ½ cup French dressing (see p. 293) Or Hain Creamy French
> 2 teaspoons Dijon mustard OR regular prepared mustard
> 1 teaspoon garlic powder
> 1 tablespoon lemon juice
> 1½ pounds turkey fillets

1. Mix all of the ingredients except the turkey to make a marinade; stir well.
2. Pour the marinade over the turkey, turning to coat all sides. Cover and refrigerate at least 2 hours, (up to 12 hours) or freeze until needed, thawing in the refrigerator.
3. Preheat the grill on high.
4. Place the fillets on the grill and reduce the heat to medium or low. Watch closely to prevent burning or flare-ups. Turn the fillets once or twice. Cook for about 30 minutes or until the center is no longer pink. Serve.

"Deviled" Turkey Fillets

TRACE OF CARBOHYDRATES   NUMBER OF SERVINGS: 3 OR 4

> 6 ounce can tomato juice (check the label for no added sugar), about ¾ cup
> 3 tablespoons Westbrae Unsweetened Un-Ketchup
> 2 teaspoons prepared mustard
> 2 teaspoons Worcestershire sauce
> 1 clove garlic, minced
> ¼ teaspoon Tabasco sauce or to taste (we prefer the mild)
> 1½ pounds turkey fillets

1. Mix all of the ingredients except the turkey to make a marinade; stir well.
2. Pour the marinade over the turkey, turning to coat all sides. Cover and refrigerate at least 2 hours, (up to 12 hours) or freeze until needed, thawing in the refrigerator.
3. Preheat the grill on high.
4. Place the fillets on the grill and reduce the heat to medium or low. Watch closely to prevent burning or flare-ups. Turn the fillets once or twice. Cook about 30 minutes, or until the center is no longer pink. Serve.

Polynesian Curry Turkey Fillets

TRACE OF CARBOHYDRATES   **NUMBER OF SERVINGS: 3 OR 4**

⅓ cup no-carb soy sauce
Zest from one orange
1 tablespoon dried onion flakes
1 tablespoon lemon juice
2 teaspoons curry powder
¼ teaspoon red cayenne pepper
1½ pounds turkey fillets

1. Mix all of the ingredients except the turkey to make a marinade; stir well.
2. Pour the marinade over the turkey, turning to coat all sides. Cover and refrigerate at least 2 hours, (up to 12 hours) or freeze until needed, thawing in the refrigerator.
3. Preheat the grill on high.
4. Place the fillets on the grill and reduce the heat to medium or low. Watch closely to prevent burning or flare-ups. Turn the fillets once or twice. Cook 20 to 30 minutes, or until the center is no longer pink. Serve.

Teriyaki Turkey Fillets

TRACE CARBOHYDRATES   **NUMBER OF SERVINGS: 3 OR 4**

½ cup no-carb soy sauce
½ cup saki or sherry cooking wine
2 cloves garlic, minced
1 teaspoon minced gingerroot OR ½ tea-
*   spoon ginger*
¼ teaspoon Liquid Smoke (optional)
1½ pounds turkey fillets

1. Mix all of the ingredients except the turkey to make a marinade; stir well.
2. Pour the marinade over the turkey, turning to coat all sides. Cover and refrigerate at least 2 hours, (up to 12 hours) or freeze until needed, thawing in the refrigerator.
3. Preheat the grill on high.
4. Place the fillets on the grill and reduce the heat to medium or medium-low. Watch closely to prevent burning or flare-ups. Turn the fillets once or twice. Cook 20 to 30 minutes, or until the center is no longer pink. Serve.

Oriental Grilled Turkey

VERY LOW CARBOHYDRATES   **NUMBER OF SERVINGS: 2**

¼ *cup peanut or olive oil*
¼ *cup no-carb soy sauce*
2 tablespoons finely minced gingerroot (½-inch slice, 1-inch diameter)
2 cloves garlic, minced
Pepper as desired
1 pound turkey fillets (2)

1. In a bowl of a small food processor or Cuisinart hand blender, place the oil, soy sauce, gingerroot, garlic, and pepper. Process until smooth.
2. Pour the marinade over the turkey and coat all sides. Place in a covered container and refrigerate at least one hour; half a day or all day would be better.
3. Heat the grill on high. Place the fillets on the grill and reduce the heat to medium. Turn the pieces to cook evenly. Cook until browned and the inside is no longer pink. Serve.

This is one of Bob's favorites!

Bombay Grilled Turkey

VERY LOW CARBOHYDRATES   **NUMBER OF SERVINGS: 2**

½ *cup lemon or lime juice (2 lemons or limes)*
¼ *cup olive oil*
1 teaspoon curry powder
½ *teaspoon cumin*
Salt and pepper to taste
1 pound turkey fillets (2)

1. Combine the lemon juice, olive oil, curry, cumin, salt, and pepper.
2. Pour the marinade over the turkey and coat all sides. Place in a covered container and refrigerate at least one hour; half a day or all day would be better.
3. Heat the outdoor grill on high. Place the fillets on the grill and reduce the heat to medium. Turn the pieces to cook evenly. Cook until browned and the inside is no longer pink. Serve.

Southwest Turkey Fillets

LOW CARBOHYDRATES   **NUMBER OF SERVINGS: 2**

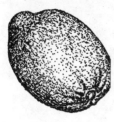

1 pound turkey fillets, cut into bite-sized pieces OR ground turkey
¾ teaspoon fajita spice blend (or mesquite seasoning)
Zest and juice from 1 lime

2 tablespoons olive oil
1 medium green pepper, cut into bite-sized chunks
½ of a medium red pepper, cut into bite-sized chunks
½ of a medium onion, cut into bite-sized chunks

Sour cream

1. Combine the turkey, spices, lime juice, and zest. Allow to marinate 1 hour, if there is time; otherwise I've cooked this immediately and it's still wonderful.
2. Put the olive oil in skillet or wok. Heat the skillet then toss in all of the ingredients except the sour cream. Stir-fry until the turkey is done, only about 5 or 10 minutes, depending on the size of the chunks.
3. Serve with a dollop of sour cream on top.

OPTIONS

- For Southwest Chicken Breasts, substitute chicken for the turkey.
- For Southwest Pork and Peppers, substitute pork loin for the turkey.

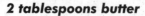

You can omit the red pepper and the dish will still taste good.

Broccoli-Turkey Stir Fry

LOW CARBOHYDRATES   **NUMBER OF SERVINGS: 3**

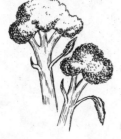

2 tablespoons butter

1½ pounds turkey fillets, cut into bite-sized chunks OR ground turkey
½ onion, chopped
1½ cup fresh broccoli, cut into bite-sized pieces
4 ounces sliced mushrooms

Back to Protein

Salt and pepper if desired

**No Carb Soy Sauce in amount desired OR
grated cheddar cheese**

1. Melt the butter in a skillet on medium heat. Add the turkey and fry until lightly browned on all sides.
2. Add the onion, broccoli, mushrooms, salt, and pepper. Cook on medium-high heat, stirring constantly until the turkey is cooked through and the broccoli is bright green and tender.
3. Serve and pass the soy sauce OR serve topped with the cheddar cheese.

OPTIONS

- Instead of the broccoli, use red or green peppers, celery, spinach, Swiss chard, or a few water chestnuts—or a combination of these up to 1½ cups.

> **This is very quick and very easy!**

Red and Green Turkey Stir Fry

NOW CARBOHYDRATES   **NUMBER OF SERVINGS: 3**

2 tablespoons butter
1½ pounds turkey fillets, cut into strips OR
    ground turkey
4 ounces sliced mushrooms
1 small onion, chopped
½ green pepper, cut into strips

½ cup red cooking wine
2 tomatoes, chopped

1. Melt the butter in a skillet on medium-high heat and quickly add the turkey, mushrooms, onion, and green pepper. Cook until the turkey is no longer pink, stirring often.
2. Pour the red wine over the ingredients in the skillet and add the tomatoes. Mix well and simmer for 5 minutes. Serve.

> **This is very quick, easy, and very good!**

Italian Turkey Stir-Fry

LOW CARBOHYDRATES **NUMBER OF SERVINGS: 4**

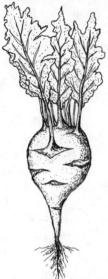

2 tablespoons butter
1½ pounds turkey fillets, cut into bite-sized chunks
8 ounces sliced mushrooms
2 or 3 ounces Canadian bacon, sliced thin, cut into strips
½ onion, chopped
½ green or red pepper, chopped
½ cup sliced black olives
½ to 1 teaspoon purchased Italian spice blend

½ cup mozzarella cheese
⅓ cup grated Parmesan cheese (optional)

1. Melt the butter in a large skillet on medium-high heat. Add the rest of the ingredients except the cheese. Stir often; cook until the turkey is browned and no longer pink inside.
2. Top with the cheeses and serve.

OPTIONS
• Pepperoni can be substituted for the Canadian bacon.
• One cup of broccoli or 1 cup of kohlrabi can be added or substituted for the green pepper and part of the mushrooms.

Ginger Turkey

VERY LOW CARBOHYDRATES **NUMBER OF SERVINGS: 3 OR 4**

2 tablespoons butter
1½ pounds turkey fillets, cut into bite-sized pieces
2 cloves garlic, minced

⅓ cup low-carb salsa
¼ teaspoon cumin
¼ teaspoon cinnamon
Gingerroot, ⅛-inch slice by 1-inch diameter, finely chopped

1. Melt the butter in a skillet on medium-high heat. Add the turkey and garlic and cook together, stirring often, until the turkey is lightly browned and no longer pink inside.
2. Add the salsa, cumin, cinnamon, and gingerroot. Simmer together about 3 minutes and serve.

Ginger Turkey with Kumquats

LOW CARBOHYDRATES   **NUMBER OF SERVINGS: 3 OR 4**

2 tablespoons olive oil
1½ pounds turkey fillets, cut into bite-sized chunks OR ground turkey
1 medium onion, thinly sliced
1½ teaspoons finely chopped gingerroot
1 green pepper, chopped
2 ribs celery, sliced (optional)
5 or 6 kumquats, thinly sliced

Soy sauce as desired

1. Heat the olive oil on medium-high heat in a skillet. Add the turkey, onion, gingerroot, green pepper, celery, and kumquats. Stir-fry until the turkey is done.
2. Serve with soy sauce.

Turkey Florentine

LOW CARBOHYDRATES   **NUMBER OF SERVINGS: 3**

2 tablespoons olive oil
4 cups fresh spinach, loosely packed
1 clove garlic, minced
Dash pepper

1½ pounds turkey fillets, cut into bite-sized chunks
Olive oil if needed

1 cup heavy cream
1 tablespoon grated Parmesan cheese
1 tablespoon white cooking wine

¼ cup slivered almonds, optional

1. Preheat the oven to 350°.
2. Heat the olive oil in a skillet on medium. Add the spinach, garlic, and pepper and stir-fry until the spinach is wilted. Place the spinach mix in a casserole dish.
3. Add more olive oil to the skillet, if needed. Cook the turkey until browned on all sides and the inside is no longer pink. Place on top of the spinach mix in casserole dish.
4. Blend together the cream, Parmesan cheese, and the wine in the skillet. Simmer on low without stirring until slightly thickened. Pour over the turkey in the casserole.
5. Place the casserole in the oven and bake for 20 minutes.
6. Sprinkle the slivered almonds on top. Return to the oven for 2 or 3 minutes to toast the almonds, then serve.

> **Developed on the author's birthday, this is really special!**

Basic Smoked Turkey Fillets

NO CARBOHYDRATES   **NUMBER OF SERVINGS 2 OR 3**

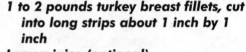

1 to 2 pounds turkey breast fillets, cut into long strips about 1 inch by 1 inch
Lemon juice (optional)
Herbs of choice (optional)
1 teaspoon cherry wood chips OR chips of choice

1. Place the wood chips in the bottom of a Camerons Stovetop Smoker. Place the drip tray and rack over the chips. Lay the turkey breast fillets on the rack. Drizzle the lemon juice over the turkey; sprinkle with the herbs, if desired.
2. Slide on the lid, leaving it barely cracked open. Place the Smoker on the largest burner on your stove; turn the heat to medium.
3. As soon as the first wisp of smoke escapes from the Smoker, close the lid and begin timing. Cooking takes 20 minutes; do not overcook.
4. Remove the smoker from the burner; serve the turkey.

OPTIONS
• This recipe also works well with chicken breasts.

Mesquite Smoked Turkey Fillets

TRACE CARBOHYDRATES   NUMBER OF SERVINGS: 3 OR 4

½ *teaspoon paprika*
½ *teaspoon cumin*
¼ *teaspoon garlic powder*
¼ *teaspoon onion powder*
¼ *teaspoon salt*
1 *to 2 pound turkey breast fillets, cut into*
   long strips about 1 inch by 1 inch

1 *teaspoon mesquite wood chips*

1. Combine the paprika, cumin, garlic powder, onion powder, and salt. Sprinkle over the turkey.
2. Place the wood chips in the bottom of a Camerons Stovetop Smoker. Place the drip tray and rack over the chips. Lay the turkey breast fillets on the rack.
3. Slide on the lid, leaving it barely cracked open. Place the Smoker on the largest burner on your stove; turn the heat to medium.
4. As soon as the first wisp of smoke escapes from the Smoker, close the lid and begin timing. Cooking takes 20 minutes; do not overcook.
5. Remove the Smoker from the stove; serve the turkey.

OPTIONS
• This recipe works well with chicken breasts.

Mom's Thanksgiving Turkey

NO CARBOHYDRATES   **NUMBER OF SERVINGS: DEPENDS ON SIZE OF TURKEY**

1 whole turkey
Butter
Sage
Salt
Onion Wedges
Water

Note: To serve for the noon meal on Thanksgiving day, start early in the morning.

1. Preheat the oven to 325°.
2. Rinse the turkey and pat dry. Remove the giblets and neck from the cavities.
3. Insert pats of butter into each cavity along with 1 teaspoon sage, ½ teaspoon salt, and onion wedges.
4. Place the turkey breast side up in a covered roasting pan. Pour 1 or 2 tablespoons melted butter over the top and close the lid. Place the turkey in the oven.
5. Periodically check the turkey. If it looks dry on the bottom, add a little water. Close the lid and return the turkey to the oven. Occasionally, baste the turkey with liquid from the bottom of roaster.
6. When the leg wiggles easily or a meat fork twists in the meat, the turkey is done. (Guidelines recommend cooking until the meat thermometer reads 180°. Place the thermometer in the inner thigh area near the breast of the turkey, but not touching the bone. Refer to the information on Meat Thermometer on p. xviii.)
7. Set the covered roaster on the counter and wait 10 minutes before carving. The meat will be moist and tender. Discard the onions and serve.

Thaw a frozen turkey in the refrigerator according to label instructions.
• Do NOT cook a frozen turkey. NEVER refreeze a partially thawed turkey.
• To ease transfer of the whole bird from the roaster to a carving platter, purchase inexpensive turkey grabbers, which are also handy during carving.
• Leftovers can be used in many ways.

Turkey with Cognac and Herbs

TRACE CARBOHYDRATES   **NUMBER OF SERVINGS: 10**

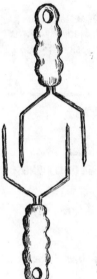

10- to 12-pound whole turkey, with or without the skin
Olive oil (if bird is skinned)
Lemon-pepper spice blend
1 large onion, cut into wedges
1 cup minced fresh parsley
2 teaspoons dried rosemary
½ carrot, sliced
½ rib celery, sliced

1 cup white cooking wine
½ cup cognac or brandy
1 cup chicken broth
½ cup Westbrae Unsweetened Un-Ketchup OR tomato sauce

1. Preheat the oven to 350°.
2. Remove the giblets and neck from the cavities; rinse the bird in cool water. Drain.
3. Use a roasting pan with a tight lid or a large cake or lasagna pan covered with heavy duty aluminum foil. Coat the pan with vegetable oil spray.
4. If your bird is skinned, rub olive oil over all surfaces.
5. Sprinkle all surfaces of a skinned or unskinned turkey with salt and lemon pepper, as desired.
6. Combine the parsley and rosemary and stuff into the cavities, along with onion wedges, carrot slices and celery.
7. In a bowl, combine the wine, cognac or brandy, broth and Un-Ketchup; pour some into each cavity and over the entire bird.
8. Put the lid on the pan tightly, or else seal tightly with foil. Place in the oven.
9. When a leg wiggles easily or meat fork twists in the meat, the turkey is done. Guidelines recommend cooking until the meat thermometer reads 180°. Place the thermometer in the inner thigh area near the breast of the turkey but not touching the bone. Refer to the information on Meat Thermometer, p. xviii and Safety Tip for Turkey on p. 209.
10. Set the covered roaster on the counter, for 10 to 15 minutes before carving. Discard vegetables. Serve the turkey with a little liquid spooned over the meat.

OPTIONS

- For a browned skin, uncover the bird for the last 30 minutes, although I've found that it browns very nicely in my covered roaster—and the meat stays very moist and tender.
- If this is too much for you to eat, just remove the meat from the bones, place in 2-cup portions in individual freezer bags, and freeze for future use. The liquid can also be frozen for use in soups.

> - **Double this recipe for a larger bird, up to 22 pounds.**
> - **Halve this recipe for half a turkey or for just a turkey breast. Since there won't be cavities to fill, just lay the raw turkey over the ingredients, skin side up.**

Turkey with Lemon and Herbs

TRACE CARBOHYDRATES — NUMBER OF SERVINGS: 10

10- to 12-pound whole turkey
1 cup lemon juice (juice from 4 lemons), plus zest
½ cup no-carb soy sauce
1 cup diced green onions plus tops (about 6)
1 tablespoon sage
1 tablespoon marjoram
1 teaspoon salt
1 teaspoon pepper

1. Preheat oven to 350°.
2. Remove the giblets and neck from the cavities; rinse the bird in cool water. Drain.
3. Use a roasting pan with a tight lid or a large cake or lasagna pan covered with heavy duty aluminum foil. Coat the pan with vegetable oil spray.
4. If your bird is skinned, rub olive oil over all surfaces.
5. Combine the lemon juice and soy sauce and pour some into each cavity and over the entire bird.
6. Combine the zest, onion, sage, marjoram, salt, and pepper and put some into each cavity; sprinkle the rest over the entire bird.
7. Cover tightly with lid or foil. Place in the oven.
8. When a leg wiggles easily or meat fork twists in the meat, the turkey is done. Guidelines say cook until the meat thermometer reads 180°. Place the thermometer in the inner thigh area near the breast of the turkey, but not touching the bone. Refer to the information on Meat Thermometers on p xviii and Safety Tips for Turkey on p 209.

9. Set the covered roaster on the counter, for 10 to 15 minutes before carving. Serve the turkey with a little liquid spooned over meat.

OPTIONS

• For browned skin, uncover the bird for the last 30 minutes, although I've found that it browns very nicely in my covered roaster—and the meat stays very moist and tender.
• If this is too much for you to eat, just remove the meat from the bones, place in 2-cup portions in individual freezer bags, and freeze for future use. The liquid can also be frozen for use in soups.

> If a whole turkey is too large for you, just cut it in half along the backbone; cook one half and freeze the other. Do this ONLY if using a fresh bird. Do NOT refreeze a thawed turkey without cooking it.
> This recipe is delicious used on a turkey breast, as well. Just halve the ingredients for a 6-pound breast.

Encore Turkey Apple Salad

LOW CARBOHYDRATES   **NUMBER OF SERVINGS: 2**

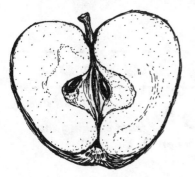

2 cups cubed cooked turkey
1 or 2 ribs diced celery
½ apple, diced
¼ cup Hellman's Original mayonnaise
½ teaspoon cinnamon
1 or 2 green onions, chopped, including tops (optional)
¼ cup pecans, toasted a few seconds under the broiler
Lettuce

1. Mix the turkey, celery, apple, mayonnaise, cinnamon, and onions together.
2. If there is time, refrigerate awhile to allow the flavors to permeate. Otherwise, serve by mounding the turkey over a lettuce leaf and top with the pecans.

OPTIONS

• Walnuts, cashews, or almonds can be substituted for the pecans.
• Cooked chicken, pork loin, or tuna can be substituted for the turkey.

Encore Turkey Curry Salad

2 cups cubed cooked turkey
2 hard-boiled eggs, diced
2 ribs celery, chopped
¼ cup black olives, sliced thin
¼ cup Hellman's Original mayonnaise
⅛ to ¼ teaspoon curry powder
Salt and pepper as desired
Lettuce
**2 tablespoons almond slivers, lightly toast-
ed under the broiler**

1. Combine the turkey, eggs, celery, olives, mayonnaise, curry powder, salt, and pepper.
2. Mound on top of a lettuce leaf. Top with almond slivers and serve.

OPTIONS

• Add a 2-ounce jar of pimentos for color.

Encore Turkey Casserole

**1½ cups broth (leftover from cooking the
turkey OR chicken Or canned)**
2 eggs

4 cups diced cooked turkey
1 cup diced celery
2 cups sliced mushrooms (about 6 ounces)
1/2 cup diced onion
Salt and pepper to taste
Parsley as garnish (optional)

1. Preheat the oven or convection oven to 350°.
2. Mix the raw eggs into the cool broth.
3. Add the turkey, celery, mushrooms, onion, salt, and pepper. Pour the mixture into a 2½-quart casserole.
4. Bake, uncovered, for 35 to 40 minutes until bubbly OR convection bake about 30 minutes.
5. Serve garnished with a parsley sprig, if desired.

Encore Turkey and Bacon in Cream

LOW CARBOHYDRATES

4 slices thick bacon

1 medium onion, sliced

3 cups diced cooked turkey
¼ teaspoon oregano (optional)
⅛ teaspoon black pepper

1 cup heavy cream
Parsley for garnish, if desired

1. Cook the bacon in a skillet until crisp. Remove the bacon to paper towels and drain off all but 1 or 2 tablespoons of the bacon grease.
2. Add the onion to skillet and cook until a little browned. Stir often.
3. Add the turkey, oregano, and pepper and toss together until blended and heated through.
4. Add the cream, stirring to blend, then bring to a boil and simmer on low without stirring until thickened.
5. Serve topped with crumbled bacon. Garnish with sprigs of parsley, if desired.

OPTIONS
- For Encore Chicken and Bacon in Cream, substitute diced cooked chicken for the turkey.

This is very fast—and delicious!

Chapter 6

FISH

& SEAFOOD

Here in rural Iowa, fish is not an everyday entree. I must wait until I'm going to town to buy groceries, which is only once every week or two, and then I must wait until my grocer has fish available—and then I take whatever that is! Consequently, we're so happy to get fresh fish that we often stick to the basics of cooking it simply—poaching, broiling, or baking it in a little butter, so as not to mar the delicate flavor.

But that would make for a slim chapter. So I've done some experimenting. Here are our favorites.

SAFETY TIPS FOR FISH AND SEAFOOD

• Keep fish and seafood chilled until cooking. Since I am a distance from the store, I generally take along an ice chest for my perishable items, like fresh fish, especially during the hot summer. (Ironically, I also use the same cooler in the winter to keep my food from freezing during our sub-zero weather!)

• Use fresh fish within 24 hours—so say the people at my store, perhaps because we're so far from a shore. If you live nearer the source, you may have more time to cook it.

• Pay attention to the smell. Fresh fish should have a mild, fresh odor or none at all. If it smells fishy, don't take it; it's probably too old. The flesh should be firm, the scales bright and close-fitting. Experts say the eyes should be clear and not glassy or sunken, but I rarely get to see the eyes where I shop.

• Thaw frozen fish in the refrigerator, and always place the fish or seafood on a pan or plate to catch any drips so that the juices do not contaminate other food. Raw juices often contain bacteria.

WHEN IS THE FISH DONE?

Fish is done when it flakes easily with a fork. The internal temperature should be 165° F, advises the Iowa State University Extension.

Basic Baked Fish

NO CARBOHYDRATES   **NUMBER OF SERVINGS: AS DESIRED**

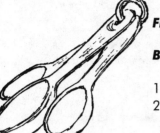

Fish of choice: cod, haddock, hake, etc.
Butter

1. Preheat the oven to 350°.
2. Place the fish on a greased ovenproof pan. Brush the fish with melted butter on all sides to prevent it from drying out. Place the fish in the oven.
3. Do Not turn the fish while baking.
4. Bake until done, or when the fish flakes easily with a fork. For fillets, it might be about 15 minutes.

OPTIONS

- Serve the fish with one of my butters or butter sauce recipes; see page 234.

> **This is very easy!**

Baked Fish &
5 Butter Sauces

NO CARBOHYDRATES   **NUMBER OF SERVINGS: 2 OR 3**

¼ cup melted butter OR olive oil
1 tablespoon lemon juice
1 teaspoon finely minced onion

1 pound pan-ready fish of choice
Paprika (optional)
Parsley for garnish (optional)

1. Preheat the oven to 350° OR to convection bake at 325°.
2. Combine the butter, lemon juice, and onion.
3. Dip or brush the butter mix all over the fish. Place the fish skin side down on an ovensafe pan, well- coated with vegetable oil spray. Pour the remaining butter over the fish.
4. Bake OR convection bake, uncovered, for 25 to 30 minutes or until done and the fish flakes easily.
5. Remove from the oven, sprinkle with paprika, and serve garnished with parsley sprigs, if desired.

Fish & Seafood   **233**

Serve the baked fish with one of the following butter sauces.

• Almond Butter Sauce:
¼ cup butter melted in small skillet + ¼ cup slivered almonds sauteed in the butter until golden; remove from the heat and add ¼ teaspoon salt and 1 teaspoon lemon juice (optional).

• Garlic Butter Sauce:
¼ cup butter melted in a small skillet + 3 cloves minced garlic sauteed in the butter until golden; remove from the heat and add a dash of salt, pepper, and ½ teaspoon lemon juice.

• Ginger Butter Sauce:
¼ cup butter melted in a small skillet + 3 cloves minced garlic + 1 teaspoon minced gingerroot sauteed in the butter until golden; remove from the heat and add a dash of salt, pepper, and 1 teaspoon lemon juice.

• Lemon Butter Sauce:
¼ cup butter + 1 ½ tablespoons lemon juice + ¼ teaspoon lemon zest + ¼ teaspoon salt + ⅛ teaspoon onion powder + dash white pepper; place all ingredients in a small pan and let it foam up but not turn brown, remove and serve.

• Caper Butter Sauce:
¼ cup melted butter + 1 tablespoon white vinegar + 2 teaspoons fresh minced parsley + 1 teaspoon capers.

• Serve the fish with one of the butters listed in the recipe for Basic Broiled Fish, page 239.

Fish Parmesan

VERY LOW CARBOHYDRATES   **NUMBER OF SERVINGS: 2**

1 pound sole fillets, or fish of choice
2 tablespoons lemon juice
Dash salt and pepper to taste

½ cup grated Parmesan cheese
⅓ cup butter, softened (microwaved for a few seconds)
2 tablespoons Hellman's Original mayonnaise OR sour cream
2 green onions, chopped, including tops

1. Preheat the broiler to high.
2. Sprinkle the lemon juice over the fish. Place in a broiler pan in a single layer and broil about 4 minutes or until opaque and the fish flakes easily with a fork.
3. Combine the Parmesan cheese, butter, mayonnaise, and onion. Spread on top of the fish and broil another minute or two, until the sauce is lightly browned. Serve.

Pecan-Coated Trout

VERY LOW CARBOHYDRATES   **NUMBER OF SERVINGS: 2**

> 1 pound fresh Canadian red trout fillets, OR
>   other mild fish
> 1 egg
> Salt to taste
> ½ cup pecan pieces
> 2 or 3 tablespoons melted butter

1. Set the oven rack down 6 inches from the broiler and preheat the broiler OR convection broiler to high heat.
2. Coat 2 individual ovenproof serving dishes OR single casserole dish with vegetable oil spray. Place the fillets skin side down in the dishes. Can coax trout into fitting into a slightly too short dish by gently pushing opposite ends of the fillet together.
3. Crack the egg into a coffee cup and beat with a fork to blend the yolk and white. Brush the egg generously on top of the fillets. Place the fish in a casserole dish.
4. Sprinkle ¼ cup of pecan pieces on each fillet.
5. Reduce the heat on broiler OR convection broiler to 350°. Place the fillets 6 inches under the broiler and leave for 10 or 12 minutes or until the fish is done—watch carefully so as not to burn the nuts.
6. Drizzle the butter the length of each fillet; return to the broiler for a few seconds and serve.

OPTIONS
• Rub the minced gingerroot on the fillet before brushing on the egg.

Trout with Almonds

VERY LOW CARBOHYDRATES   **NUMBER OF SERVINGS: 4**

> 2 pounds fresh Canadian red trout fillets or
>   steaks OR other mild fish
> 2 eggs
> Salt and pepper as desired
> 1½ cups ground pork rinds
>
> 2 tablespoons butter
> ½ cup slivered almonds
> 2 tablespoons Worcestershire sauce
> 1 tablespoon lemon juice
> 1 tablespoon minced fresh parsley (optional)

Fish & Seafood   **235**

1. Preheat the oven OR convection oven to 350°.
2. Coat the broiler rack with vegetable oil spray.
3. Crack the eggs into a coffeecup and beat with a fork to blend the yolk and white.
4. Place the pork rinds in a small pie plate and blend in the salt and pepper.
5. Brush the egg generously on the fish, then roll the fish into the ground pork rinds. (Note: Discard any unused pork rind.) Place on broiler rack. Bake in the oven about 30 minutes OR convection bake about 25 minutes, or until done and fish flakes easily. Watch carefully so the coating does not burn.
6. In a small skillet, melt the butter. Add the almonds and brown slightly. Add the Worcestershire sauce and lemon juice, stir together, and heat through. Pour the almond mix over the fish, sprinkle the minced parsley on top, and serve.

Fish Florentine

VERY LOW CARBOHYDRATES   **NUMBER OF SERVINGS: 2**

1 tablespoon butter
1 to 2 cups chopped fresh spinach, packed

¼ cup Hellman's Original mayonnaise
1 egg yolk
¼ cup finely diced onion
2 tablespoons grated Parmesan cheese
2 teaspoons lemon juice
Dash nutmeg, freshly ground if possible
Dash salt, if desired

2 tablespoons melted butter
1 pound fish fillets, cod OR halibut OR other mild fish

¼ cup additional grated Parmesan cheese

1. Set oven rack down 6 inches from broiler and preheat broiler OR convection broiler to high heat.
2. Melt the butter in a skillet and add the spinach. Stir-fry until the spinach is wilted. Remove from the heat.
3. Add the mayonnaise, egg yolk, onion, Parmesan cheese, lemon juice, nutmeg, and salt to the skillet. Mix well.
4. Place the fish on an ovenproof pan coated with vegetable oil spray, skin sides down. Brush melted butter on top. Place the fish under the broiler and reduce the heat to 350°. Remove when the fish is opaque and lightly browned.

5. Spread the spinach mixture over each fillet. Return to the broiler to heat through.
6. Top with additional Parmesan cheese, place under the broiler a few seconds more, and serve.

Baked Fish with Pork Rind Coating

TRACE CARBOHYDRATES   NUMBER OF SERVINGS: 2

1 pound fish (I've used quite a range, from mahi-mahi to pollock)
1 egg OR 4 tablespoons melted butter OR ½ cup buttermilk or cream
1 cup ground pork rinds (or more, if needed)
Dash salt
¼ cup melted butter (omit if using the butter, above)

1. Preheat the oven to 350°.
2. Dip the fish in the beaten egg and then into the ground pork rinds. (Note: Discard any unused pork rind.) Place on a roasting rack over a baking dish OR use the broiler rack and pan.
3. Sprinkle the fish with salt; drizzle with butter.
4. Bake for about 30 minutes until opaque and flaky and serve.

• We used to purchase frozen pollock in 10-pound boxes as a school fundraiser. Although it is not my favorite fish, this is my favorite recipe for it.
• All the coatings are good; the buttermilk is our favorite, followed by the butter. The buttermilk has 6.5 grams of carb; however, much of the milk is left behind in the dipping pan, to our cats' delight!

Herbed Baked Fish

1 pound fish, fresh OR thawed and drained

¼ cup melted butter OR 1 egg OR ½ cup buttermilk or cream

¾ cup ground pork rinds
¼ cup grated Parmesan cheese
½ teaspoon basil
½ teaspoon oregano
½ teaspoon salt
¼ teaspoon garlic powder

1. Preheat the oven to at 350° OR convection bake at 325°.
2. Combine the pork rinds, Parmesan cheese, basil, oregano, salt, and garlic powder.
3. Dip the fish in the melted butter and then into the pork rind mixture. Discard any unused pork rinds. Put on a rack in a baking pan. Drizzle any remaining butter over the fish OR melt a little more for this.
4. Bake OR convection bake for 30 minutes or until the fish flakes easily with a fork. Serve.

Basic Broiled Fish & 9 Butters

NO CARBOHYDRATES   NUMBER OF SERVINGS: AS DESIRED

Pan-ready fish of choice
Butter or olive oil
Salt and pepper
Parsley for garnish (optional)

1. Preheat the broiler to high.
2. Dip the fish in butter or oil. Sprinkle with salt and pepper, if desired.
3. Place the fish skin side down on a broiler that's been coated with vegetable oil spray. Place the broiler pan about 4 inches under the heat. Broil about 10 minutes or until browned—watch closely. Do NOT turn fish.
4. Serve the fish garnished with parsley sprigs, if desired.

OPTIONS
- Serve the fish with a little fresh-squeezed lemon.
- Serve the fish with one of the following butters:

- Anchovy Butter:
¼ cup softened butter + 2 teaspoons anchovy paste (mash anchovies with a fork).

- Lemon-Parsley Butter:
¼ cup softened butter + ¼ cup fresh minced parsley + 1 ½ tablespoons lemon juice + pinch lemon zest.

- Lemon-Basil Butter:
¼ cup softened butter + ½ teaspoon grated lemon peel + ½ teaspoon lemon juice + ¼ teaspoon basil.

- Lime Butter:
¼ cup softened butter + ½ tablespoon lime juice + pinch lime zest.

- Tarragon Spice Butter:
¼ cup melted butter + 2 tablespoons tarragon vinegar + 1 tablespoon freshly minced parsley + several drops Worcestershire sauce.

- Cajun Butter:
¼ cup softened butter + ½ teaspoon oregano + ¼ teaspoon cumin + ⅛ teaspoon thyme + dash red pepper.

- Fennel Butter:
¼ cup softened butter + 1 teaspoon fennel seed, crushed + ½ teaspoon lemon juice + dash pepper.

- Italian Butter:
¼ cup softened butter + 1 tablespoon grated Parmesan cheese + ½ teaspoon Italian blend seasoning + ½ teaspoon garlic powder.

- Parmesan Butter:
¼ cup softened butter + 1 tablespoon grated Parmesan cheese + 1 teaspoon parsley flakes + ¼ teaspoon garlic powder.

- Serve the fish with one of the butter sauces listed with the recipe for Baked Fish, page 233.

Poached Halibut

TRACE CARBOHYDRATES   NUMBER OF SERVINGS: 3

Boiling water
1½ pounds halibut steak OR fish of choice
4 peppercorns
2 teaspoons lemon juice
½ bay leaf

1. Place a tray in a fish poacher and place the fish on the tray. Because the poacher is long and narrow, I straddle the pan over two smaller burners rather than center it on a large burner.
2. Cover the fish with the boiling water poured down the side of the poacher. Add the peppercorns, lemon juice, and bay leaf.
3. Gently simmer on low for about 10 minutes, or until the fish is done. Do not overcook.
4. Pull up the poacher rack, remove the fish and serve. Garnish with lemon slices or parsley sprigs, if desired.

Generally speaking, poaching doesn't work as well for the slimmer fish fillets because they tend to be too delicate and fall apart even with the gentlest simmer. Poaching works best with fish steaks, or whole fish, or really thick fish fillets.

Steamed Fish

NO CARBOHYDRATES   NUMBER OF SERVINGS: 3 OR 4

1 to 2 pounds halibut, salmon, OR fish of
choice, fillets, steaks, OR pan-dressed fish
Water

1. Pour water into the fish poacher-steamer about 1½ inches deep (it should not touch the fish). Place the poacher so it straddles two burners. (Note: The rack in the fish poacher reverses; when placed upside down in the poaching pan, it becomes a fish steamer.)
2. Place the steamer rack in the water; turn both burners on high to bring the water to a boil.
3. Place the fish on the rack; reduce the temperature to a low boil. Cover tightly with the poacher lid. Allow to steam for 5 or 10 minutes or longer, until the fish is done and flakes easily.

OPTIONS
• Serve with a butter or butter sauce, if desired.

This couldn't be easier!

240   *Back to Protein*

Poached Ocean Pike

VERY LOW CARBOHYDRATES   **NUMBER OF SERVINGS: 3 TO 6**

Water
1 teaspoon salt
1 or 2 pounds ocean pike OR fish of choice

1 or 2 tablespoons vinegar
½ large onion, sliced
½ to ¾ cup chopped celery
1 large lemon, sliced, (discard the ends)
1 bay leaf

1. Place 1 to 1 1/4 inches of water in the fish poacher. Add salt. Bring the water to a boil.
2. Place the fish on the poacher rack and insert the rack into the poacher. Immediately reduce the heat to a low gentle simmer.
3. Drizzle vinegar over the fish. Place the onion and celery on top and then cover all with the lemon slices. Place a bay leaf in the water.
4. Cover and simmer until the fish is just done. Do NOT overcook.
5. Pull up the poacher rack, remove the fish, and serve. Garnish with additional lemon slices or parsley sprigs, if desired.

The reason for the variation in the amount of fish is that the fish poacher will hold up to 2 pounds comfortably, with the same amount of water and other ingredients.

Italian Fish

LOW CARBOHYDRATES   **NUMBER OF SERVINGS: 2 OR 3**

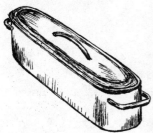

1 pound fish of choice, skin removed

15 ounce can tomato sauce
1 tablespoon minced fresh parsley
½ teaspoon dried basil
¼ teaspoon oregano
Dash black pepper

¾ cup shredded mozzarella cheese
Parsley for garnish

1. Preheat the oven to 350°.
2. Coat a covered casserole dish just large enough to hold the fish snugly in a single layer with vegetable oil spray. Place the fish in the casserole.

3. Combine the tomato sauce, parsley, basil, oregano, and black pepper. Pour over the fish.
4. Bake, covered, for 40 minutes or until the fish is tender and flakes easily.
5. Sprinkle the fish with mozzarella and return to the oven, uncovered, until the cheese melts and is lightly browned.
6. Serve garnished with parsley sprigs.

OPTIONS
- Add a few mushroom slices and/or green pepper strips to the tomato sauce.
- Top the cheese with slivered almonds before returning to oven.

Grilled Rainbow Trout

VERY LOW CARBOHYDRATES   **NUMBER OF SERVINGS: 2**

1 pound rainbow trout fillets OR red snapper steaks OR other fish of choice

¼ cup olive oil
2 tablespoons lemon juice
½ teaspoon salt
¼ teaspoon Worcestershire sauce
⅛ teaspoon pepper
Dash Tabasco sauce (we use the mild)
Paprika

1. Preheat the outdoor grill on high heat.
2. Coat the hinged wire grill rack generously with vegetable oil spray. Place the fish inside the grill rack and close securely.
3. Combine the olive oil, lemon juice, salt, Worcestershire sauce, pepper, and Tabasco sauce. Brush generously onto both sides of the fish through the grill rack. Sprinkle with paprika.
4. Place the hinged grill rack on the grill; close the lid as much as possible, and reduce the heat to medium.
5. After 4 minutes, baste the top side of the fish with the remaining liquid, flip the hinged grill rack, and baste the other side.
6. Remove the fish from the grill when done, perhaps another 4 minutes; fish will flake easily and look opaque.
7. Serve garnished with lemon wedges, if desired.

Seafood Kabobs

Shrimp, scallops or a firm fish like halibut,
*   salmon or tuna*
Onion, cut into 1 inch chunks
Melted butter

(Note: If using bamboo skewers, soak for 30 minutes in water so they do not burn. OR use metal skewers.)

1. Preheat the grill OR broiler.
2. Thread the seafood and onions on the skewers. Brush on a heavy coat of butter.
3. Place the skewers on the grill OR broiler, basting often with additional butter to prevent the fish/seafood from drying out or sticking to the grill. Watch closely, turning after 2 or 3 minutes. Total cooking time will be only 6 or 7 minutes. Fish will look opaque throughout when done.
4. Remove from the heat and serve.

OPTIONS

- Instead of using plain butter, use an Herbed Butter Basting Sauce: ¼ cup melted butter + 1 tablespoon fresh minced parsley + ½ teaspoon lemon juice + ¾ teaspoon dried herb(s) of your choice, (basil, oregano, thyme). Brush on skewers.

Sweet Peppers and Salmon

VERY LOW CARBOHYDRATES   **NUMBER OF SERVINGS: 2 OR 3**

1 pound salmon fillets
1 quarter of a green sweet pepper
1 quarter of a red sweet pepper
1 quarter of a yellow sweet pepper
Dash garlic powder OR garlic salt
Dash thyme

1. Preheat the grill on high.
2. Place the fillets skin side down on a piece of heavy duty aluminum foil. Cut the peppers into slices and cut the slices into 1-inch lengths, place on top of the salmon. Sprinkle with a generous dash of garlic powder or garlic salt and a dash of thyme. Seal the foil by bringing opposing sides together and folding over several times. Roll and pinch the ends.
3. Place the foil package on the grill and reduce the heat to medium. Close the lid and cook for about 12 minutes. Fish will be done and peppers will be tender-crisp.
4. Open the foil and serve. (Warning: The escaping steam can burn your skin!)

OPTIONS

- Place the foil packages on a cookie sheet in a 350° oven for about 30 minutes.

This is quick, easy, and colorful.

Baked Salmon with Dill

VERY LOW CARBOHYDRATES   **NUMBER OF SERVINGS: 2 OR 3**

About 1½ pounds salmon steaks OR fillets
½ cup white cooking wine
6 green onions, chopped, including tops
½ teaspoon dried dill weed
¼ teaspoon mace
¼ teaspoon pepper

Lemon slices for garnish (optional)

1. Preheat oven to bake at350° OR convection bake at 325°.
2. Coat an oven-proof dish with vegetable oil spray. Place the salmon in dish the in a single layer, skin side down if using fillets.

3. Pour the wine over the salmon and then top with the onion, dill weed, mace, and pepper.
4. Bake, uncovered, for 35 minutes OR convection bake for about 30 minutes until the fish fillet flakes easily and looks opaque or until a knife can be easily inserted in the steak.
5. Serve garnished with lemon slices, if desired.

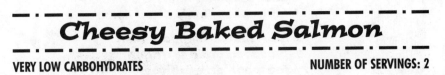

Cheesy Baked Salmon

VERY LOW CARBOHYDRATES   **NUMBER OF SERVINGS: 2**

1 pound salmon steaks OR fillets
Dash salt and pepper if desired
1 tablespoon finely diced onions
½ cup shredded cheddar cheese
¼ cup sour cream

1. Preheat oven to bake at 350° OR convection bake at 325°.
2. Coat an oven-proof dish with vegetable oil spray. Place the salmon in the dish in a single layer, skin side down if using fillets. Sprinkle with salt and pepper, if desired (I usually omit this).
3. Top with the onion and then the cheddar. Spoon small dollops of the sour cream on top of the cheese.
4. Bake for 30 minutes OR convection bake for about 25 minutes until the fish flakes easily and looks opaque or until a knife can be easily inserted in the steak. Serve.

OPTIONS

This recipe works well with other types of fish.

It's not every day that we have access to fresh salmon here in farm country. We love the flavor of plain salmon so much that I am always reluctant to experiment to create new recipes that might disappoint us, but this dish is truly exceptional!

Salmon with Tarragon Butter

TRACE OF CARBOHYDRATES　　　　　　　　　　　　　　**NUMBER OF SERVINGS: 2**

1 pound salmon fillets OR steaks
1 tablespoon finely diced onion

2 tablespoons melted butter
½ teaspoon dried tarragon
½ teaspoon dried chives
¼ teaspoon dried parsley
1½ teaspoons Dijon mustard

1. Preheat broiler OR convection broiler on high heat.
2. Coat an oven-proof dish with vegetable oil spray. Place the salmon in the dish in a single layer, skin side down if using fillets. Sprinkle onion on top.
3. For Tarragon Chive Butter, combine the butter, tarragon, chives, parsley, and Dijon mustard. Spread the mixture on top of the salmon.
4. Broil OR convection broil on the top rack about 4 minutes on high heat for 2 minutes, then turn the broiler off and leave the salmon in another 2 minutes. Salmon should flake easily and look opaque.
5. Serve garnished with a sprig of fresh parsley, if desired.

OPTIONS

- Instead of the tarragon butter, use Lemon Parsley Butter: 2 tablespoons softened butter + 1 teaspoons lemon juice + ¼ teaspoon lemon zest + 1 ½ teaspoons minced fresh parsley + dash salt and pepper.

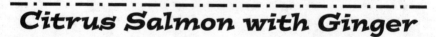

We're not big tarragon fans, but this dish is outstanding!

Citrus Salmon with Ginger

LOW CARBOHYDRATES　　　　　　　　　　　　　　**NUMBER OF SERVINGS: 2**

1 pound salmon fillets or steaks OR halibut
or other mild fish

Zest from 1 lemon
Juice from 1 lemon
1 tablespoon olive oil
1 tablespoon minced gingerroot (½ inch
slice 1-inch in diameter) OR 1-teaspoon
ginger

2 tablespoons melted butter

1. Place the salmon in an oven-proof dish that has been coated with vegetable oil spray.
2. Make a marinade from the zest, lemon juice, olive oil, and gingerroot, using a hand blender.
3. Pour the marinade over the salmon. Cover and refrigerate 2 hours or overnight.
4. Lower the rack to 6 inches below the broiler. Preheat the broiler to high heat.
5. Drizzle the butter over the salmon; place the salmon under the broiler and reduce the heat to 350°. Broil until the salmon flakes easily and looks opaque and the butter is a little browned—6 to 10 minutes, depending on the thickness of the salmon.
6. Serve with additional lemon slices, if desired.

OPTIONS

- Substitute a lime for the lemon.

Smoked Fish

NUMBER OF SERVINGS: 2

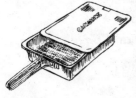

1 pound cod OR other fish fillets
½ teaspoon wood chips of choice
1 to 2 tablespoons lemon juice
Dill weed, if desired
Black pepper, as desired

Sour cream, if desired

1. Place the wood chips in the bottom of a Camerons Stovetop Smoker. Place the drip tray and rack over the chips. Coat the rack with vegetable oil spray. Lay the fish on the rack. Drizzle the lemon juice over the fish and sprinkle with dill and pepper.
2. Slide on the lid, leaving it barely cracked open. Place the Smoker on the largest burner on your stove; turn the heat to medium.
3. As soon as the first wisp of smoke escapes from the Smoker, close the lid and begin timing. Allow 15 minutes, remove the fish and serve with a dollop of sour cream.

OPTIONS

- After the fish has smoked, remove the lid and cover the fish with 1 or 2 tablespoons of melted butter. Then put the Smoker under the broiler a few seconds until the fish is slightly browned.

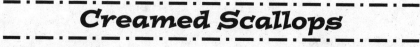

Creamed Scallops

LOW CARBOHYDRATES   **NUMBER OF SERVINGS: 2**

2 tablespoons butter
1 pound fresh scallops, rinsed in cold water
    and drained

1 cup heavy cream
¼ teaspoon salt
Dash black pepper

1. Melt the butter in a medium skillet and add the scallops. Stir-fry until done; scallops will be opaque white inside.
2. Add the cream, salt, and pepper and simmer on low without stirring until the sauce is thickened.
3. Serve the scallops with the sauce.

Easy Shrimp Scampi

VERY LOW CARBOHYDRATES   **NUMBER OF SERVINGS: 2 OR 3**

2 tablespoons melted butter
2 cloves garlic, minced

1 pound shrimp, peeled and deveined

¼ cup white cooking wine
1 tablespoon lemon juice
⅛ teaspoon salt
Dash pepper

1 tablespoon minced fresh parsley
Lemon wedges (optional)

1. Melt the butter in a skillet. Add the garlic, and saute for 1 minute, until lightly browned. Add the shrimp and saute for 1 minute.
2. Add the wine, lemon juice, salt, and pepper. Continue sauteeing until the sauce is reduced and shrimp are bright pink.
3. Sprinkle with parsley and serve garnished with lemon wedges, if desired.

Shrimp & Mushroom Stir Fry

LOW CARBOHYDRATES **NUMBER OF SERVINGS: 2**

> 1 to 2 tablespoons butter
> ½ pound shrimp, (peeled, deveined and rinsed)
> 4 ounces sliced mushrooms
>
> ½ cup sour cream
> 1½ teaspoons soy sauce
> ⅛ teaspoon paprika
>
> ⅓ cup shredded Monterey Jack blend cheese

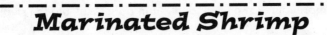

1. Melt the butter in a skillet and stir-fry the shrimp and mushrooms for about 5 minutes on medium.
2. Combine the sour cream, soy sauce and paprika and pour over the shrimp. Reduce the heat and simmer on low until well-heated.
3. Top with the cheese and serve.

Marinated Shrimp

VERY LOW CARBOHYDRATES **NUMBER OF SERVINGS: 2 FOR MAIN COURSE
5 OR 6 FOR APPETIZERS**

> 1 pound small cooked, peeled, deveined shrimp
> ¼ cup olive oil
> ¼ cup soy sauce
> ¼ cup cooking sherry
> 1 tablespoon lemon juice
> ½ teaspoon purchased Italian spice blend
> ¼ teaspoon ginger
> ¼ teaspoon garlic salt

1. Combine all of the ingredients in a bowl; cover and refrigerate for 3 to 4 hours.
2. Stir, and serve cold.

OPTIONS
• After marinading, shrimp can be skewered and grilled OR broil until lightly browned.

> Since most of the marinade is left behind, this recipe actually is close to being no-carb.

Broiled Tuna Steak

NO CARBOHYDRATES   **NUMBER OF SERVINGS: 2**

1 tablespoon butter

1 pound tuna steaks OR fillets
2 tablespoons vermouth
Salt and pepper as desired

1. Preheat the broiler on high heat.
2. Choose an ovenproof pan only a little larger than the tuna laid out in a single layer. Put butter in the pan and place the pan under the broiler a few seconds until the butter is melted.
3. Tilt the pan to spread the butter all over the bottom. Place the tuna in the pan; if using fillets, place the skin side down.
4. Remove the skin from the outside of the tuna, if using steaks; the skin is really tough. Also, remove any dark purple or brown flesh at the edge. It's edible, but unsightly. Place the tuna in the pan.
5. Drizzle the vermouth over the tuna; sprinkle on salt and pepper as desired.
6. Place the tuna under the broiler for about 3 minutes. Remove and drizzle 1 tablespoon butter over the tuna and return to the broiler for 2 to 3 more minutes, or until done. If in doubt, cut into the steak; it should be cooked through and opaque, but not overdone.
7. Serve.

OPTIONS
- Just before serving, top the tuna with snipped chives OR chopped green onion, including tops.

Basic Tuna Salad

VERY LOW CARBOHYDRATES   **NUMBER OF SERVINGS: 1**

6 ounce can tuna, drained
¼ to ½ cup chopped vegetables, total, chosen from:
- cauliflower
- celery
- water chestnuts
- green bell pepper or sweet red pepper
- pimento

2 tablespoons diced green onion, including tops OR 1 tablespoon finely diced onion
1½ teaspoons lemon juice
¼ teaspoon prepared mustard

⅛ teaspoon curry powder
2 or 3 tablespoons Hellman's Original mayonnaise
2 tablespoons slivered almonds, toasted a few seconds under broiler (optional)

Lettuce
Shredded cheddar

1. Combine the tuna, vegetables, onion, lemon juice, mustard, curry, and mayonnaise. Mound on top of lettuce, if desired.
2. Sprinkle on some cheddar cheese, if desired. Serve topped with the toasted almond slivers.

OPTIONS
- Sprinkle a little lemon zest over the finished salad.
- Substitute 1 cup of diced cooked turkey for the tuna—great!

> Flavors will permeate throughout the salad much better if it's refrigerated a few hours, though I often eat it right after making it and it still tastes wonderful!

Hot or Cold Tuna Salad

TRACE OR VERY LOW CARBOHYDRATES   NUMBER OF SERVINGS: 1

6 ounce can tuna, drained
1 hard-boiled egg, chopped (optional)
1 tablespoon chopped green pepper (optional)
1 or 2 tablespoons chopped green olives with pimento (optional)
1 or 2 tablespoons Hellman's Original mayonnaise
¼ to ½ cup shredded cheddar cheese OR cheese of choice

Mix ingredients together and serve.

OPTIONS
- Serve cold tuna on a lettuce leaf.
- Serve this dish hot—just pop in the microwave for 30 seconds or until heated through.

> This is very fast!

Mexican Tuna Salad

2 6-ounce cans tuna, drained
¼ to ½ cup shredded cheddar cheese
¼ cup sliced green olives stuffed with
    pimento
1 or 2 green onions, chopped, including
    tops
3 to 4 tablespoons Hellman's Original may-
    onnaise OR sour cream
¼ teaspoon chili powder (or more, to taste)
⅛ teaspoon garlic powder (or more, to
    taste)
Paprika

Lettuce leaves
Diced avocado (optional)
Tomato slices (optional)

1. Combine the tuna, cheddar cheese, olives, onion, mayonnaise, chili
   powder, and garlic powder. Sprinkle with paprika.
2. Serve as is, cold, or mound on lettuce leaves garnished with avocado and tomato.

OPTIONS
• Substitute black olives for the green.

Cashew Tuna Salad

6- or 9-ounce can tuna, drained
¼ cup diced celery
1 to 2 tablespoons finely diced onion
Salt and pepper as desired
2 tablespoons Hellman's Original mayon-
    naise OR sour cream

Lettuce (optional)
¼ cup cashews, raw if possible, toasted a
    few seconds under the broiler

1. Mix together the tuna, celery, onion, salt, pepper, and mayonnaise.
2. To serve, mound on top of lettuce, if desired, and top with the toasted cashews.

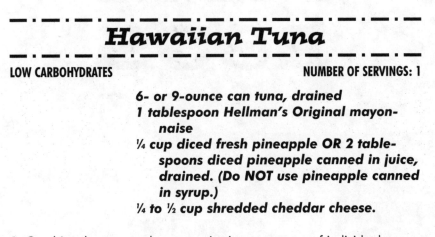

Hawaiian Tuna

LOW CARBOHYDRATES   **NUMBER OF SERVINGS: 1**

6- or 9-ounce can tuna, drained
1 tablespoon Hellman's Original mayonnaise
¼ cup diced fresh pineapple OR 2 tablespoons diced pineapple canned in juice, drained. (Do NOT use pineapple canned in syrup.)
¼ to ½ cup shredded cheddar cheese.

1. Combine the tuna and mayonnaise in an oven-proof individual serving casserole dish.
2. Place the pineapple on the tuna.
3. Sprinkle the cheddar cheese over all. Microwave for 30 seconds or until heated through and the cheese is slightly melted OR place under the broiler for a few seconds. Serve.

OPTIONS
• Substitute canned sliced mushrooms, drained, for the pineapple.

Chapter 7

EGGS

Eggs—what a high-quality protein at a very low price! Rich in nutrients, egg yolks are one of the few food sources of vitamin D. Now that we're past the cholesterol-scare nonsense, we can eat a diet rich in eggs. In fact, Bob has them for breakfast nearly every morning.

You'll notice that I include eggs in many of my animal protein recipes. This is for the nutrition boost as well as for eggs' inherent cooking qualities: they keep burgers from falling apart, they hold crumb coatings in place, and they work as a thickener in casseroles.

Farm-fresh eggs just can't be beat, and the same neighbor who raises free-range chickens also provides us with wonderful eggs. We buy 6 dozen at a time, delivered fresh to our door. Thanks, Terry!

EGG INFO

• To avoid the greenish ring that sometimes forms around the yolk of hard-boiled eggs, be sure to run cold water over them as soon as the cooking time is up.

• There is no difference between eggs with brown and white shells. We use both.

• Store eggs with the large end up.

SAFETY TIPS FOR EGGS

Salmonella—a bacteria that causes food poisoning—can grow inside fresh, unbroken eggs. To avoid problems:

- Cook eggs until the yolk and white are firm, not runny.
- Scramble eggs to a firm texture.
- Don't use recipes in which eggs remain raw or only partially cooked.
- Either destroy cracked eggs, or use them promptly by cooking them thoroughly.

EGG STORAGE TIPS

• Eggs stored in their shells in a refrigerator at 40°F will keep about 3 weeks. (The American Egg Board says they'll keep refrigerated in their carton at least 4 to 5 weeks past their expiration date)

• Hard-boiled eggs will keep in the refrigerator one week.
• Don't freeze fresh or hard-cooked eggs.

(Information from the Iowa State University Extension.)

Hard-boiled Eggs & 2 Butters

TRACE OF CARBOHYDRATES   **NUMBER OF SERVINGS: AS DESIRED**

Eggs
Cold water

1. Place the eggs in a saucepan so they are somewhat crowded. Cover with cold tap water. Turn the burner on high; when the water comes to a boil, cover the pan and reduce the heat to a low simmer for 15 minutes.
2. Remove the lid. Carry the pan to the sink and fill with cold tap water. Dump the water and fill with cold water again. Repeat.
3. To separate eggs from the shell, remove one egg from the cold water, dry it off, and gently tap it on the counter until the entire surface is cracked. Then roll the egg gently in your hands. Slip a spoon under the shell, and it will slide right off the egg.

OPTIONS

- Freshly cooked hard-boiled eggs are delicious sliced and sprinkled with salt and pepper and topped with a pat of butter while still warm. OR, if necessary, heat a few seconds in the microwave.
- Top warm hard-boiled eggs with one of the following butters:

Chili Herb Butter:
¼ cup softened butter + ⅛ teaspoon thyme + ⅛ teaspoon oregano + ⅛ teaspoon chili powder.

Mustard Butter:
3 tablespoons softened butter + 1 teaspoon prepared mustard.
SEE ALSO other butters and butter sauces on pages 66–68, 234, 239, 243, and 246.

> While you're at it, boil more eggs than you need. They come in handy as snacks or as additions to other dishes. Store hard-boiled eggs in the refrigerator. To distinguish hard-boiled eggs from fresh raw eggs, draw a face on the shell with a pencil or a magic marker. OR spin the egg. A hard-cooked egg spins easily, but a raw egg wobbles.

Stuffed Eggs

TRACE OF CARBOHYDRATES   NUMBER OF SERVINGS: AS DESIRED, MAKES 12

*3 slices bacon (I prefer thick-sliced hickory-
  smoked bacon)*
6 hard-boiled eggs, sliced lengthwise
*1 to 2 tablespoons Hellman's Original may-
  onnaise*
1 tablespoon finely chopped fresh parsley
¼ teaspoon salt
⅛ teaspoon black pepper

Paprika
Sliced green olives stuffed with pimentos
Lettuce

1. Cut the bacon strips in half and fry in a medium skillet until very crisp.
   Cool on a paper towel, then crumble into small bits.
2. Carefully remove the yolks from the eggs; place in a bowl. Add the
   bacon, mayonnaise, parsley, salt, and pepper; blend well.
3. Mound the yolk mixture onto the egg whites, sprinkle with paprika,
   then press an olive slice onto each. Serve on a bed of lettuce.

These make great appetizers.

Deviled Eggs

TRACE OF CARBOHYDRATES   NUMBER OF SERVINGS: AS DESIRED, MAKES 12

6 hard-boiled eggs, sliced lengthwise
*2 to 3 tablespoons Hellman's Original may-
  onnaise*
2 teaspoons lemon juice OR vinegar
1 teaspoon Worcestershire sauce
¾ teaspoon prepared mustard
⅛ teaspoon salt
⅛ teaspoon pepper

Paprika
Lettuce (optional)

1. Carefully remove the yolks from the eggs; place in a bowl. Add the
   remaining ingredients; blend well.
2. Spoon the yolk mixture onto egg whites OR use a pastry tube to fill;
   sprinkle with paprika, and serve on a bed of lettuce.

• Add some chopped parsley or finely minced meat or fish to the yolk mixture.

Egg Salad Supreme

VERY LOW CARBOHYDRATES   **NUMBER OF SERVINGS: 2**

> **8 hard-boiled eggs, chopped**
> **1 ⅓ cup shredded cheddar cheese**
> **⅓ cup finely diced celery**
> **3 tablespoons coarsely diced green olives with pimentos**
> **2 or 3 tablespoons Hellman's Original mayonnaise**
> **Salt and pepper, as desired**
> **Lettuce**

1. Combine all of the ingredients except the lettuce.
2. Place the lettuce on salad plates and mound the egg salad on top. Serve.

OPTIONS
• Garnish with slices from an additional olive OR a wild violet flower.

This makes a great low-carb substitute for egg salad sandwiches!

Hard-Boiled Eggs with Cream Cheese Sauce

VERY LOW CARBOHYDRATES   **NUMBER OF SERVINGS: 2**

> **8 hard-boiled eggs, peeled and sliced**
>
> **3 ounces Philadelphia Cream Cheese**
> **⅓ cup heavy whipping cream**
> **3 tablespoons grated Parmesan cheese**

1. Place the cream cheese, whipping cream, and the Parmesan cheese in a 2 cup Pyrex measure. Microwave on medium for 3 or 4 minutes, or until the sauce is smooth. Stir after 2 minutes.
2. Pour over the eggs and serve.

• Sprinkle a little paprika on top.

> • **An egg slicer is inexpensive and fast and easy to use!**
> • **For diced eggs, run the egg through the slicer twice, once horizontally and once with the egg vertically.**

Hard-Boiled Eggs with Welsh Rabbit Sauce

LOW CARBOHYDRATES   **NUMBER OF SERVINGS: 2**

8 hard-boiled eggs, peeled and sliced

2 cups shredded cheddar cheese
⅓ cup heavy cream
¼ teaspoon mustard
¼ teaspoon Worcestershire sauce
⅛ teaspoon salt
Dash pepper
Parsley for garnish

1. Heat the cheddar cheese in a 4-cup Pyrex measurer in the microwave until almost melted. Add the cream, mustard, Worcestershire sauce, salt, and pepper.
2. Pour over warm eggs and serve, garnished with parsley, if desired.

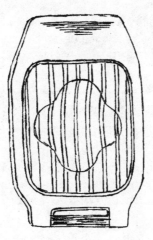

Creamed Eggs and Asparagus

LOW CARBOHYDRATES   **NUMBER OF SERVINGS: 3**

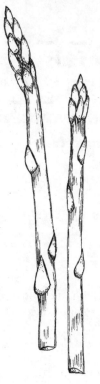

1½ cups asparagus, cut into 1-inch lengths
1 cup heavy whipping cream
1 teaspoon Dijon mustard
Salt and pepper to taste

9 or 12 hard-boiled eggs, removed from shells and diced
Paprika

1. Steam or cook the asparagus in a little water until tender; drain thoroughly.
2. Return the asparagus to a saucepan and add the cream, Dijon mustard, salt, and pepper. Simmer on low until thickened.
3. Add the eggs to the cream mixture and heat through.
4. Sprinkle each serving with paprika.

OPTIONS

- Try adding a little diced ham to this dish; top with a sprinkle of shredded cheddar cheese.

> I invented this dish when we were adding on to our house and were living without a kitchen for almost six months; cooking was done using only a hot plate, a microwave, and an outdoor grill. We ate this often in the spring and early summer when our asparagus was ready to be picked.

Creamed Ham & Eggs

LOW CARBOHYDRATES   **NUMBER OF SERVINGS: 2**

8 hard-boiled eggs
½ cup finely chopped ham OR Canadian bacon OR 3 to 4 slices of bacon, crumbled
3 or 4 finely chopped green onions, including tops
½ teaspoon Worcestershire sauce
½ teaspoon prepared mustard (I prefer Dijon) OR ½ teaspoon dry mustard

1 cup heavy cream
1 teaspoon chicken bouillon granules
Dash white pepper

1 or 2 tablespoons finely chopped parsley

1. In a medium saucepan, mix together the eggs, ham or bacon, onions, Worcestershire sauce, and mustard. Cover the pan and put it on the lowest heat setting.
2. Put the heavy cream, bouillon, and white pepper into a small skillet. Simmer on low until thickened.
3. Pour the cream over the egg mixture, sprinkle with the parsley, and serve.

OPTIONS
- Sliced green olives stuffed with pimento make a tasty garnish. So do fresh radish slices.
- Add 2 ounces of red pimento to the egg mixture for color and flavor.

Egg & Encore Chicken Scramble

VERY LOW CARBOHYDRATES   **NUMBER OF SERVINGS: 2**

6 eggs
2 green onions, chopped
2 tablespoons minced fresh parsley
½ teaspoon celery seed
¼ teaspoon tarragon
Salt and pepper to taste

1 to 2 tablespoons butter

1 cup chopped cooked chicken

1. Crack the eggs into a bowl; stir the yolks and whites together with a fork. Add the onions, parsley, celery seed, tarragon, salt, and pepper.
2. Melt the butter in a skillet on medium heat. Pour the egg mixture over the butter. Top with the chicken. As the eggs solidify on the bottom, stir the pan.
3. When cooked through, garnish with pieces of additional parsley, if desired, and serve.

OPTIONS
- Instead of the chicken, you can substitute almost any kind of leftover meat: ham, turkey, pork roast, etc.

This is colorful when garnished also with thin tomato slices.

Eggs   **261**

Basic Omelette

3 large eggs
1 tablespoons water
¼ teaspoon salt (optional)
⅛ teaspoon pepper (optional)

1½ to 2 tablespoons butter
About ½ cup filling; choose from:
  diced ham; crumbled bacon; sliced
  mushrooms; shredded or grated cheeses;
  chopped onion; cooked spinach, leftover
  cooked meat, fish, seafood, or poultry
  diced fine; a little chopped green pep-
  per or tomato; green chilies
OR Make
  • Spinach Omelette: spinach + Parmesan
    cheese + dash nutmeg
  • Avocado Omelette: diced avocado +
    chicken + chives

1. Crack the eggs in a bowl and beat with a fork. Add the water and the salt and pepper; stir.
2. Melt the butter on medium-high heat in a 7- or 8-inch nonstick skillet. Swirl it around the bottom and sides of the pan; the butter should be hot enough to foam, but do NOT allow butter to brown.
3. Pour the egg mixture all at once in the center of the pan and reduce the heat to medium-low. Scrape the cooked egg from the outside towards the center with an inverted pancake turner on four sides of the skillet. Allow the uncooked egg to run to the bottom of the pan.
4. Aim the handle of the omelette pan towards your waist. When the surface of the egg looks creamy and not runny, it's time to put the filling on the left half of the omelette. Slide a pancake turner under the outer edges of the omelette to make certain it isn't stuck to the bottom. Then fold the right half of the omelette over the left half with the pancake turner.
5. Holding the handle, flip the pan upside down onto a serving plate. Enjoy!

OPTIONS

• For Herb Omelettes, add the following to the egg mixture before cooking:

¼ teaspoon freshly minced parsley + ⅛ teaspoon oregano or basil + ¼ teaspoon chives (optional) OR

1 tablespoon minced fresh parsley OR

1 tablespoon minced fresh parsley + ⅛ teaspoon dried dillweed.

• For Tangy Omelettes, add a drop or two or of Worcestershire sauce to the egg mixture before cooking.

Don't worry if you have trouble making a perfect omelette at first; you can always stir the eggs and the filling together and call it scrambled eggs!
Choose a nonstick skillet with very low rounded sides for an omelette pan, so the eggs cannot become lodged where the sides join the bottom and so you can easily loosen the omelette with a pancake turner. Some people reserve a special pan just for omelettes.

Basic Scrambled Eggs

VERY LOW CARBOHYDRATES   **NUMBER OF SERVINGS: 1**

2 large eggs
2 tablespoons cream or milk
Dash salt and pepper, if desired

1 to 2 tablespoons butter
Parsley, for garnish (optional)

1. Crack the eggs in a bowl and beat with a fork. Add the water and the salt and pepper; stir.
2. Melt the butter in a 8- to10-inch nonstick skillet on medium-high heat. Swirl it around the bottom and sides of the pan; the butter should be hot enough to foam, but do NOT allow the butter to brown.
3. Pour the egg mixture into the center of the pan, reduce heat the to medium-low, and shake the pan with one hand. When the eggs have solidified on the bottom of the pan, scrape across the cooked egg with an inverted pancake turner from time to time. The eggs are done when no visible liquid remains and the eggs are soft curds.
4. Serve garnished with a sprig of parsley, if desired.

OPTIONS
• Add any of the following to the egg mixture before cooking:
diced ham; crumbled bacon; sauteed mushrooms; shredded cheeses; chopped onion; cooked spinach, leftover cooked meat, fish, seafood, or poultry diced fine; a little chopped green pepper or tomato; green chilies, capers, horseradish
• Herbs and spices that can be added to the egg mixture include:
basil, chili powder, chives, curry, dill, Fines herbes, hot pepper sauce, marjoram, dry mustard, paprika, parsley, savory, tarragon, thyme OR

try spinach + Parmesan cheese + dash nutmeg OR

diced avocado + chicken + chives OR

¼ teaspoon freshly minced parsley + ⅛ teaspoon oregano or basil + ¼ teaspoon chives (optional) OR

1 tablespoon minced fresh parsley OR

1 tablespoon minced fresh parsley + ⅛ teaspoon dried dillweed OR

a drop or two or Worcestershire sauce

> **You can easily multiply this recipe, using up to about a dozen large eggs in one large skillet, but do not increase the butter over 2 tablespoons; use the least amount necessary to coat the bottom of the skillet. Crack all the eggs into a bowl, beat, then add all the cream and any desired additions before cooking.**

Egg and Spinach Frittata

LOW CARBOHYDRATES **NUMBER OF SERVINGS: 2 OR 3**

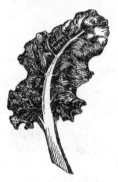

8 eggs
1 teaspoon dried parsley
Dash pepper
Dash of nutmeg (freshly ground, if possible)

2 tablespoons butter
3 cups fresh spinach leaves, chopped OR
   Swiss chard leaves, chopped, with the ribs removed
¾ cup chopped green onion, including tops
1 large clove garlic, minced

1. Break the eggs into a medium bowl and beat with a fork until the whites and yolks are blended. Add the parsley, pepper, and nutmeg. Set aside.
2. Preheat the broiler or convection broiler to high.
3. Melt the butter in an ovenproof skillet; add the spinach, onion, and garlic. Stir-fry on medium heat until spinach leaves are wilted.
4. Add the egg mixture and cook on the stovetop without stirring on medium-low heat until the bottom is lightly browned.
5. Place under the broiler for about 1 minute until the top is lightly browned.
6. Sprinkle the sesame seeds on top of the eggs and return to the broiler for a few seconds until lightly toasted—watch carefully so the sesame seeds do not burn. Serve.

OPTIONS

- I've often substituted fresh Swiss chard for the spinach because the chard is in season much longer. Remove the stalks from two leaves and chop and cook the same as the spinach.

> **This makes a wonderful breakfast dish that doesn't take much time.**

Eggs "Pizza"

6 eggs
5 or 6 sliced black olives
3 tablespoons grated Parmesan cheese
½ to 1 teaspoon purchased pizza spice
    blend
1 clove minced garlic (optional)

2 ounces pepperoni slices OR Canadian
    bacon
4 ounces sliced mushrooms (or more)

1 cup shredded mozzarella cheese

1. Preheat the broiler or convection broiler to high.
2. Crack the eggs into a bowl and stir with a fork until the yolks and whites are blended. Add the olives, Parmesan cheese, pizza spice, and garlic. Stir together and set aside.
3. Stir-fry the pepperoni or bacon and mushrooms in an ovenproof skillet on medium heat until the mushrooms are done. The fat from the meat should be enough; if not, add a little butter.
4. Pour the egg mixture into the skillet on top of the meat. Cook without stirring, until the bottom of the eggs are just lightly browned; the tops will not be done.
5. Transfer the skillet to the broiler a short while; remove when the eggs are just barely browned on top.
6. Top the eggs with the mozzarella cheese and return to the broiler for a few seconds until the cheese is melted and lightly browned. Serve.

OPTIONS
- Add ½ cup chopped green pepper with the mushrooms.

This is great served with tender young asparagus stems that are lightly steamed and topped with a pat of butter.

Crustless Spinach Quiche

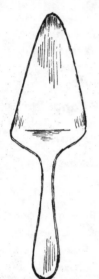

2 to 2½ cups chopped fresh spinach
3 green onions, thinly sliced OR 1 medium onion, chopped
⅔ cup shredded Swiss or mozzarella cheese
⅔ cup shredded cheddar cheese

9 eggs
1½ cups half-and-half OR heavy cream
½ teaspoon salt
½ teaspoon pepper
⅛ teaspoon nutmeg
⅛ teaspoon garlic powder
Parmesan cheese

1. Preheat the oven to 350°.
2. Butter a quiche dish or a deep pie plate. Place the spinach in the bottom. Top with the Swiss and cheddar cheeses.
3. Crack the eggs into a medium bowl and add the cream, salt, pepper, nutmeg, and garlic powder. Pour into the quiche dish.
4. Bake for 30 minutes. Pull the rack out of the oven and sprinkle Parmesan cheese on top. Bake for another 15 minutes and serve.

OPTIONS

• I often use Swiss chard leaves picked fresh from the garden. For this dish, I cut out the rib and then chop the greens. An excellent alternative to the spinach!

This makes a wonderful breakfast when entertaining guests!

Chapter 8

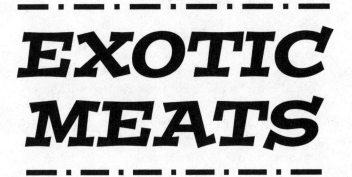

EXOTIC MEATS

TIPS FOR COOKING EXOTIC MEATS

As people return to a protein-based diet, interest is returning to eating the meats our forebears hunted and ate of necessity to survive. Now considered exotic, these meats are being farm-raised and can be ordered for a taste treat.

My thanks to Ryan Larsen, Manager of Seattle's Finest Exotic Meats, Inc. for helping me learn about cooking the exotics. Thanks also to Randy Redig, Rudy Flege, and Bill Brenny for their contribution of meats for testing.

Alligator

Alligator is a versatile meat, as far as the reptiles go. Its history is long, and it comes mainly from the Southern states where it is harvested. Its taste can be described as a cross between pork and fish, perhaps due to its diet of fish, turtles, and occasional birds, or perhaps due to what must be a shared muscle lubricant that works like an antifreeze for cold-blooded creatures. The best meat comes from a cylindrical tube inside the tail; this meat is white and is the most tender and tasty. Meat from the body is darker, stronger in taste, and tougher in texture—somewhat similar to pork shoulder roast.

Well-suited to a simmering sauce, lemon flavors and spicy flavors fit the fishy taste of the gator well. The easiest way to cook it is to simmer it for 25 to 30 minutes in the sauce of your choice, or try one of the beef recipes and make it into a soup or stew.

Alligator meat can also be ground and often is mixed with beef or pork; then, it is cooked much like hamburger.

Antelope

Although they look like deer, antelope are actually part of a family that includes goats and oxen. The meat is finely grained and mild tasting, similar to venison. The key to working with any of the exotic red meats is to use olive oil; it's essential to replace the moisture you would otherwise be cooking out.

Cut the antelope into ½-inch strips and marinate the meat in olive oil for 2 to 6 hours with your favorite spices before cooking. Ryan prefers using a well-heated cast-iron skillet with a generous splash of olive oil. He likes the heat high and the cooking time low, and he keeps the meat "dancing in the pan" for 1 to 1½ minutes.

Buffalo

Similar to beef, but sweet and rich with a somewhat "bolder" taste, buffalo is high in protein and has about half the fat of beef. It takes less buffalo to fill you up due to the density of the meat and the high protein that your body craves, so allow less meat per serving. The buffalo industry is definitely growing, and it's not uncommon to find it in restaurants these days. Because of its growing popularity, Midwestern farmers are looking at buffalo as an alternate livestock for income.

Buffalo can be used in any recipe that calls for beef. Because it is low-fat, cook buffalo steaks slowly on low heat and only to rare or medium rare. Seasonings can include garlic salt and lemon-pepper OR cut the steak into ½-inch strips and marinate in olive oil for 2 to 6 hours, as with the antelope. Then cook it at a higher heat for a short while.

For roast cuts, try making a stew in a Crock-Pot or cook in a pressure cooker. If baked, the oven should be set 50° cooler oven than for beef, and the internal temperature should reach 170°.

For stews, the meat can be cooked to well-done, because of the liquid. The meat will be tender.

Caribou

Closely related to the reindeer, caribou offers meat that is finely grained and resembles veal or antelope—which is close to venison, which is close to elk. If you haven't sampled them, the taste distinctions are difficult to describe; just think how you'd describe the taste difference between an orange and a tangerine to someone who hasn't tried either.

For cooking, apply the exotic red meat rules: olive oil, high heat, low cook time. Expect a great-tasting piece of meat if cooked as instructed.

Cervina

New Zealand red deer—see Venison.

Cobra

Cobra is like calamari in taste and texture. But if it is not cooked properly, it can be tough and rubbery. It's best simmered in a sauce for about 45 minutes, which will make it delicate and tender like chicken.

Duck

The Muscovy duck is farm-raised in northern California and has considerably more fat and larger breasts than its wild counterpart. They are generally harvested at 2 to 3 pounds and taste a bit like liver; they can be stringy in texture.

Duck is good roasted, or in soups.

Elk

Another alternative livestock Midwestern farmers are just starting to consider raising is elk. The second largest member in the deer family, elk offers meat that is very dark, coarsely grained, and the sweetest of the deer family—with a mild flavor.

Elk sausages and burgers are fun to cook and taste great. Cook elk steak by the exotic red meat rules: olive oil, high heat, low cook time. You can also cook elk with the same recipes that use venison.

Frog legs

As the old cliché goes, frog legs really do taste something like chicken crossed with fish. Legs can have the salty taste of clams when pan-fried in oil or take on a fishy taste when cooked with moisture. Either way, they're good, and it's easy to see why the French like them so much.

Cook frog legs like you would any chicken recipe. Chicken—think chicken—and you'll have a great meal with no prior experience.

Goose

Somewhat like well-done beef, goose is all dark meat. Because of the fat, you should prick the skin every inch or so to release the fat during baking. Even so, the meat is very lean at about 7 percent, but lacks the high protein count of most of the exotics.

To cook, the big roasting birds all seem to follow the same game plan when it comes to roasting bags: Dutch ovens, open ovens, whatever.

Toulouse Goose

Harvested before it is nine months old weighing between 8 to 12 pounds, the Toulouse goose is more tender, more supple, and has more meat that its wild counterpart. But it's still dark meat, still goose, and still cooked the same.

Kangaroo

This animal is one of Ryan's personal favorites; he describes kangaroo meat as a cross between venison and a good beef steak, with a sweetness about it. Low in fat, high in protein, with a great flavor, this meat shouldn't be overlooked.

To cook, follow the exotic red meat rules. Or substitute kangaroo for venison in your favorite recipe.

Lamb

Australian lamb is said to be far superior to both the New Zealand lamb and the American lamb. Both the Australian lamb and the New Zealand lamb are rare in the US, which makes them exotic meats.

Cook as you would any lamb.

Ostrich and Emu

What a great meat! This is one of the best exotics to begin with if you are accustomed to eating beef, poultry, and pork. Similar to beef in taste and texture, but lower in fat and higher in protein, ostrich has the best feed-to-weight ratio of any land animal in the world.

During the farm crisis of the 1980s, I suggested using our empty cattle facilities for ostriches, only to get one of those "You're crazy, woman!" looks from my husband. A neighbor did go into it, experienced success, and now has a herd of 200 head.

Ostrich and emu are close in flavor, but some people think of emu meat as more moist, and it is—by 1 percent: emu has 3 percent fat while ostrich has 2 percent. But it's all in how it's cooked. There is no shrinkage in ostrich when cooked.

Recipes and methods for veal work well for ostrich. Because of its dark red meat, ostrich follows the exotic meat rule: olive oil, high heat, low cook time. Highly recommended!

Pheasant

One of the most popular of the game birds, pheasants grow wild here in Iowa and we have flocks on our farm, but they are not native to the U.S. In an effort to develop them as game birds, every county in Iowa was sent a pair of pheasants via the railroad. As a young lad, close family friend, Lute Thornton (born in the 1880s) was present at their introduction. Lute's father had the responsibility for receiving the pheasants and releasing the first pair in Pocahontas county. The male birds are quite beautiful and are targeted for hunting during a limited season, leaving the smaller, plainer-looking hens to produce chicks the following spring.

As a child, I had a pet pheasant that had been orphaned; we were told we were the first to successfully raise a chick in captivity. He lived in our basement. I would sing to him each day and he would warble back. Eventually, we released him on our farm and he would roost high on a limb outside the farmhouse. Our worries about his ability to adapt were unfounded; he even brought a mate to roost on the branch with him.

I was raised on pheasant; my father hunted them, dressed them, and my mother cooked them. The pheasant we ate growing up was tasty, but we had to beware of biting down hard on the buckshot. Once when I was bumped to first class on a plane returning from Europe, I was startled to discover buckshot in my farm-raised pheasant under glass!

Pheasant tastes different from chicken, although the breast offers wonderful white meat and the leg and thigh meat is darker, like a chicken. Ryan says that farm-raised pheasant has a subtle, delicate flavor, often with a discernible trace of apple. A whole-dressed pheasant can weigh between 2 and 3 pounds.

The meat is low in fat and can dry out easily when cooked. Ryan recommends frying pheasant quickly at a high temperature in plenty of oil. Serve immediately; it toughens as it stands.

Quail

This bird has red meat with a delicate texture and a sweet nutty flavor. Quail is often stuffed with a ground meat due to its small size of 5 to 6 ounces with only a few ounces, of breast meat. Supposedly you're to allow 2 quail per person, but Ryan suggests 4 is more likely to satisfy a male appetite. Quail is very elegant and impressive at a nice dinner.

Baking or roasting quail is recommended. Brush often with butter and with broth, to keep it from drying. You can roast them with a half-slice of bacon draped over each breast.

Rabbit

Farm-raised rabbit has a lean, slightly sweet meat with a closely textured flesh that has virtually no fat and is very high in protein. It's an alternative to chicken because it's a white meat, and diners often wouldn't know it wasn't chicken if you didn't tell them.

The thighs and legs are usually roasted. The saddle, or the front part, is best stewed.

Ryan prefers to coat the meat with olive oil and fry it in a cast-iron skillet with more olive oil. To keep it from becoming dry, he says, think olive oil.

Rattlesnake

Ryan says the old 'tastes like chicken' belief is true with rattlesnake. In fact, he calls it "velvet chicken" because it's so perfectly grained.

If the meat has the bones in, you'll need to cook the rattler in chicken broth and any herbs or spices you desire—or don't desire—for about 20 minutes. Then you need to debone the cooked meat. Tedious, yes; but worth it, yes! This gives you a pile of rattlesnake meat that you can do just about anything with—pick your favorite chicken recipe. Ryan says it's also suited for fine chili seasoning.

Our son, Chris, recently had rattler that was cooked, whole, on an outdoor grill, with no seasoning. He ate it by picking the meat off the bones, and said it was quite good, like chicken.

Scottish Grouse and Partridge

Both animals weigh about one pound. Grouse is an extraordinary delicacy with dark flesh; it's best roasted or braised. Partridge is succulent, with a pronounced gamey flavor; it takes well to grilling and sauteeing. Both are lean.

Squab (Pigeon or Rock Dove)

This meat is succulent but still has some earthy taste to it, which pleases many of the squab fans. Rich, dark, and very delicate, the average squab weighs about 14 ounces, enough to serve one person.

Cook squab medium rare so that the juices run pink and the meat remains slightly rosy and moist.

Snapping Turtle

With the texture of frog legs or lobster, the four legs and the tail are the dark meat; the neck and back straps are the white meat. Die-hard fans say there are seven—count 'em—seven colors in the turtle meat, and it is the next best thing to heaven.

Turtle can be pan-fried, in the usual "exotic" way: lots of olive oil, high heat, low cooking time. It's best to marinate or soup this meat, says Ryan. It goes well with lemon or Cajun flavors.

Venison

One is Ryan's favorite of all the exotics, he calls venison "the candy of meats"—so good he dreams about it! He says a package of venison flank steak can make friends faster than a stack of 100 dollar bills! Venison is the low-fat meat that will knock your socks off.

We have herds of wild deer on our farm that cost us a lot of money, as they help themselves to the crops in our fields. They've also become less afraid and are taking a toll on my vegetable and flower gardens; they do significant damage to my orchard, my pine tree wind breaks, and my ornamental crab apple trees; they'll kill saplings; and they've even eaten my weeping willow to the ground several times. Years ago, I totaled my first car when a deer jumped out of the ditch and we collided—I still have the antlers. They're lovely animals and beautiful to watch as they float over our fences, but all in all we'd rather not have them here. So we don't mind when our friends hunt them, especially when they share some of the meat!

I have a century-old recipe for deer meat that starts out "First, get your deer!" Although everyone I know here in Iowa eats game deer, Ryan says farm-raised deer is better because it lacks the gamey flavor. The New Zealand red deer is the best venison on the market.

Follow the red meat cooking rule: lots of olive oil, high heat, low cooking time. Ryan likes his meat plain, straight out of the skillet with the steam still rising—this is heaven!

Wild Boar

Any pork fan will immediately recognize the rich, sweet, deep pork flavor that they crave, but wild boar is leaner and deeper red than pork. When harvested young, it's tender without any effort. Ryan recommends this meat to anyone, exotic meat fan or not.

Wild Boar needs to be cooked well to rid it of the chance of trichinosis as with pork. The chops are great grilled, the same as pork chops with your favorite flavors. The tenderloin is incredible, says Ryan, and Bob and I both agree.

Bear (Black)

Bear meat reflects the animal quite well—it is tough! Ryan says any animal that knocks down trees is going to be tough, wouldn't you agree?

The burger is fantastic with a texture somewhat like buffalo, but with a definite bold flavor behind that easy-going burger texture. Ryan says the steak is best for stewing. Both should be cooked well, because bear can carry trichinosis, too.

Llama

If you like the inviting flavor of veal, you will really go for this one, says Ryan. The burgers are terrific; the steaks superb and very lean.

Llama an be grilled or pan-fried, using the exotic red meat rule. Ryan suggests cooking the burgers until they're gray all the way through.

Grilled Alligator Tail

LOW CARBOHYDRATES   **NUMBER OF SERVINGS: 3**

> *1 pound alligator tail*
> *Salt and pepper*
> *Lemon juice*
> *Butter*

1. Place the alligator meat on heavy aluminum foil. Sprinkle with salt and pepper; coat with lemon juice and butter. Seal the foil.
2. Cook on the grill on medium heat, turning often, about 20 or 30 minutes. Do not overcook.
3. Serve with additional lemon-butter.

OPTIONS

- After you've sprinkled the meat with salt and pepper and coated it with lemon juice and butter, pan-fry it on high heat in butter. This works best with the meat cut into strips, rather than leaving steak whole, so you can stir-fry the meat. Sprinkle with additional lemon juice and serve with lemon butter.
- Cook the meat in Camerons Stovetop Smoker.

Basic Grilled Bison Steak

TRACE OF CARBOHYDRATES   **NUMBER OF SERVINGS: AS DESIRED**

> *Bison steaks: rib eye, T-bone, New York strip*
> *(less tender cuts need to be marinated)*
> *Seasonings of choice: garlic, salt, olive oil,*
> *lemon-pepper*

1. Preheat the grill to high.
2. Rub the steaks with seasonings of choice (see above).
3. Place the steaks on the grill and reduce the heat to medium (325°).
4. Turn the steaks with tongs, not a fork, to keep the juices sealed inside.
5. Cook bison to either rare or medium and serve.

COOKING TIMES

1"-thick Rare: 6 to 8 minutes/side Medium: 8 to 10 minutes/side
1½"-thick Rare: 8 to 10 minutes/side Medium: 10 to 12 minutes/side
2"-thick Rare: 10 to 12 minutes/side Medium: 14 to 18 minutes/side

> **Information courtesy the National Bison Association**

Grilled Bison Burgers

> 1⅓ pounds lean ground bison
> ¼ cup finely chopped onion
> 2 tablespoons Westbrae Unsweetened Un-
> Ketchup
> 2 teaspoons dry mustard
> 2 teaspoons oregano
> 1 teaspoon garlic salt
> ½ teaspoon black pepper

1. Preheat the grill on high.
2. In a medium bowl, combine the meat, onion, Un-Ketchup, mustard, oregano, garlic salt, and pepper. Mix until blended. Form into patties.
3. Place the burgers on the grill, close the lid, and reduce the heat to medium. Cook 7 minutes per side or to desired degree of doneness; ground meat should always be cooked to medium-well, with no pink inside. Serve.

OPTIONS

• Additional condiments include Hellman's Original mayonnaise, mustard, dill pickles, additional Westbrae Unsweetened Un-Ketchup, lettuce, thin slices of onion, thin slices of tomato.

Recipe courtesy the National Bison Association

Bison Kebobs

> 2 tablespoons olive oil
> 2 cloves garlic, minced
> 3 tablespoons balsamic vinegar
> 2 teaspoons basil
> 2 teaspoons bay leaf
> ¼ teaspoon black pepper
> 1 pound bison round roast, whole OR cut
> into 1-inch pieces
> 1 onion, cut into 1-inch chunks
> 1 green pepper, cut into 1-inch chunks
> 12 mushrooms

1. Combine the marinade ingredients in a food processor or blender until smooth OR shake in a tightly covered glass jar. Pour into a glass container and add the bison pieces. Cover and refrigerate for 4 to 8 hours.
2. Preheat the grill on high heat.
3. Remove the meat from the marinade and thread onto 6 skewers with the onion, green pepper, and mushrooms. Brush marinade over the vegetables and meat on the skewers.
4. Place the skewers on the grill and reduce the heat to low. Cook until the meat is medium rare, basting occasionally with leftover marinade during the first half of the cooking process. Serve.

• Remember low 'n slow. Overcooked buffalo meat will bring you the same results of other overcooked meats—something that resembles roofing shingles.
• "With buffalo, what you see is what you get. There is little shrinkage due to fat. Bison rivals the finest beef available. Once you've tried it, you'll come back for more."—Comments and recipe from the Wooden Nickel Buffalo Farm.

Savory Bison Oven Roasted Meat Balls

LOW CARBOHYDRATES NUMBER OF SERVINGS: 3 OR MORE AS DESIRED, MAKES 24 MEAT BALLS

1 pound ground bison
½ cup finely chopped mushrooms
⅓ cup finely chopped red onion
1 egg, beaten
2 cloves garlic, minced
1 teaspoon salt
1 teaspoon ground black pepper
1 teaspoon Italian seasoning
Dipping sauce (recipe below)

1. Preheat the oven to 400°.
2. In a medium bowl, combine all of the ingredients. Mix until well-blended. Form into 24 meatballs about the size of a large walnut.
3. Coat a jelly roll pan with vegetable oil spray. Place meatballs in the pan.
4. Roast, uncovered, in the oven for 10 minutes.
5. Serve with the dipping sauce.

Thyme Vinaigrette Dressing

TRACE OF CARBOHYDRATES   AMOUNT: ABOUT ⅔ CUP

½ cup olive oil
2 tablespoons red wine vinegar
1 tablespoon Dijon OR Grey Poupon mustard
2 teaspoons soy sauce
½ teaspoon dried thyme
¼ teaspoon black pepper
1 clove garlic, minced

Place all of the ingredients in a small container with a tightly-sealing lid and shake well OR use a Cuisinart hand blender with blade.

Lemon Dressing

TRACE OF CARBOHYDRATES   AMOUNT: ABOUT 1 CUP

¼ cup olive oil OR oil of choice
2 or 3 tablespoons grated Parmesan OR Romano cheese
2 tablespoons lemon juice
¼ teaspoon lemon zest
¼ teaspoon black pepper

Place all of the ingredients in a small container with a tightly-sealing lid and shake well OR use a blender with blade.

OPTIONS
• Add ½ teaspoon of your favorite dried herb seasoning blend.

Coriander Dressing

TRACE OF CARBOHYDRATES   AMOUNT: ABOUT 1 CUP

¾ cup olive oil
3 tablespoons tarragon vinegar
1 tablespoon water
1½ teaspoons coriander
1 teaspoon Dijon mustard

Dipping Sauce

⅔ cup Hellman's Original mayonnaise
⅓ cup Dijon mustard
3 tablespoons chopped green onions

Combine in a small bowl; stir to blend. Serve with the meatballs.

Recipe courtesy the National Bison Association

Bison Fajitas on a Stick

VERY LOW CARBOHYDRATES   **NUMBER OF SERVINGS: 4**

¼ cup tequila OR lemon juice
2 tablespoons minced fresh cilantro leaves
4 cloves garlic, minced
½ teaspoon grated lime zest
1 tablespoon lime juice
½ teaspoon salt
½ teaspoon red pepper flakes
¼ teaspoon black pepper

1½ pounds bison steak, cut into 1-inch strips
8 wooden skewers, soaked in water 30 minutes OR metal skewers

1. Combine the tequila or lemon juice, cilantro leaves, garlic, lime zest and juice, salt, and peppers. Pour into a resealable plastic bag. Add the bison; seal the bag and turn to coat the meat thoroughly with the marinade. Place in the refrigerator for 1 hour or overnight.
2. Preheat the grill or broiler on high.
3. Remove the meat from the marinade and thread onto the skewers. Grill or broil to desired doneness and serve.

Recipe courtesy the National Bison Association

Deer Burgers

TRACE CARBOHYDRATES   **NUMBER OF SERVINGS: 4 OR 5**

> 1 pound smoked venison sausage (no sugar
>   added)
> 1 pound ground beef
> 1 egg
> 1 to 2 tablespoons lemon-pepper season-
>   ing blend

1. Preheat the broiler to high.
2. Combine all of the ingredients. Shape into patties; place the patties
   on the broiler rack.
3. Place the broiler 4 or 5 inches under the heat for 5 minutes, turning
   once. Serve.

OPTIONS
- Substitute smoked beef sausage for the venison.

Easy Deer Chops

TRACE OF CARBOHYDRATES   **NUMBER OF SERVINGS: AS DESIRED**

> 1½ inch thick venison chops
> Italian salad dressing, bottled, OR use my
>   Italian Dressing recipe, (see page 296)

1. Marinate the venison in the Italian dressing 6 to 8 hours in the refrigerator.
2. Preheat the broiler to high.
3. Broil 2 inches from the heat—3 minutes per side for rare, 4 minutes
   per side for medium, or 5 minutes per side for well-done.
4. Remove from the heat and serve.

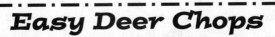

Do not overcook, or the meat will be tough.

Marinade for Smoked Deer

LOW CARBOHYDRATES   **NUMBER OF SERVINGS: AS DESIRED**

1½ cups red cooking wine
½ cup red wine vinegar
½ cup oil
½ cup chopped onion
1 teaspoon oregano
1 clove garlic, minced

Deer meat: steaks, roast, or cut of choice
Bacon strips
Pecan chips

1. Mix all of the ingredients except the meat and chips to make the marinade; pour over the deer meat and marinate for 3 days.
2. Remove from the marinade. Cover the meat with strips of bacon.
3. Place pecan chips in the bottom of a Camerons Stovetop Smoker, about 1 teaspoon per 2 pounds meat. Cover the chips with the drip tray, topped with the rack. Place the deer on the rack. Cover with the lid or make a tightly-sealed tent of heavy aluminum foil.
4. Place the smoker on a burner on medium heat OR on an outdoor grill on medium heat. Cook meat about 25 minutes per pound, or to desired doneness.

Recipe courtesy of Camerons Stovetop Smoker.

Deer Stew

VERY LOW CARBOHYDRATES   **NUMBER OF SERVINGS: 3 OR 4**

1½ pounds venison round steak, sliced thin
    into 2 inch strips
Salt and pepper

1 tablespoon butter
1 cup broth
1 teaspoon prepared hot and spicy mustard
¼ cup sour cream at room temperature
Dash Kitchen Bouquet

2 tablespoons butter
1 large onion, sliced

Back to Protein

1. Generously sprinkle the salt and pepper on the steak. Set aside.
2. Melt the butter in a skillet. Add the broth, the mustard, and the sour cream. Bring to a boil, then reduce the heat. Add a dash of Kitchen Bouquet.
3. In another skillet, melt 2 tablespoons butter. Add meat and onion, and brown quickly on high heat. Discard the onion and add meat to the sour cream sauce. Cover and keep hot 20 minutes, without simmering. Serve.

Deer Sausage Stew

LOW CARBOHYDRATES   **NUMBER OF SERVINGS: 3 OR 4**

1 tablespoon butter
About 1½ pound venison summer sausage, cut into ¼ inch slices and each slice quartered
½ cup onion, chopped
½ cup green pepper, chopped
¼ teaspoon thyme
¼ teaspoon oregano
1 small bay leaf
2 cups canned whole tomatoes + juice
1 cup beef broth

1. Melt the butter in a large skillet. Add the remaining ingredients and bring to a boil.
2. Reduce the heat and simmer for about 30 minutes. Serve in bowls.

OPTIONS

• Taste a slice of the summer sausage before using it in this recipe. If it tastes salty (ours did), simmer the sausage in a little water for 5 to 10 minutes. Then pour off the water and use the sausage in this recipe.

Our neighbor supplied us with the sausage, from deer he hunted on our land. Thanks, Randy!

Aunt Nell's Wild Duck

NO CARBOHYDRATES   **NUMBER OF SERVINGS: 2**

One wild duck
Salt
Celery, chopped
Onion, chopped

1. Clean the duck; wash and drain. Sprinkle salt inside and out.
2. Stuff the duck with celery and onion to draw out the wild taste.
3. Place in a covered baking pan. Bake at 375° for 1 hour. Uncover and bake about 1 more hour, or until brown. (It should be done enough that the juices should not run red, but not so done that the meat is falling off the bone.)
4. Discard the celery and onion and serve.

Aunt Nell's Canadian Goose

TRACE CARBOHYDRATES   **NUMBER OF SERVINGS: 6 OR 7**

6- to 7-pound wild Canadian goose
Onion
Celery
Nuts of choice: pecans, almonds, or walnuts

2 tablespoons butter
8 ounces sliced fresh mushrooms
1 cup chicken broth

1. Preheat the oven to 500°.
2. Clean, wash and dry the goose. Stuff with the onion, celery, and nuts.
3. Bake, uncovered, for 30 minutes.
4. Reduce the heat to 350°, cover, and bake for 1 hour.
5. Melt the butter in a skillet; cook the mushrooms for about 5 minutes. Pour in the broth, simmer about 5 minutes. Pour broth mixture over the goose and bake another hour, or until well-done. Serve.

Dijon Smoked Game Birds

NO CARBOHYDRATES   **NUMBER OF SERVINGS: AS DESIRED**

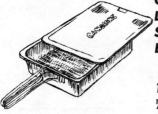

Game birds (pheasant, etc.)
Dijon mustard
Salt and pepper
Bacon strips (especially if wild; if
    domestic, can omit)

1 tablespoon oak wood chips
½ tablespoon pecan woods chips

1. Split the birds and brush with Dijon mustard, salt, and pepper.
2. Place the wood chips in the bottom of a Camerons Stovetop Smoker. Place the drip tray and rack over the chips. Lay the birds on the rack.
3. Slide on the lid if it fits over the birds. Otherwise, make a foil tent over the top of the birds, tightly sealing all around. If necessary to make a seam in the foil, be certain it is also tightly sealed.
4. Place the Smoker on the largest burner on your stove; turn the heat to medium.
5. Cooking takes about 25 minutes per pound.
6. Remove the foil tent. Place the smoker under the broiler a few seconds until the skin is lightly browned. Serve.

Recipe courtesy Camerons Stovetop Smoker.

Ostrich Burgers

VERY LOW CARBOHYDRATES   **NUMBER OF SERVINGS: 3**

1 teaspoon olive oil
1 clove garlic, minced
2 tablespoons finely diced onion

1 pound ground ostrich meat
1 teaspoon salt
½ teaspoon freshly ground black pepper

1. Place the olive oil in a skillet and saute the garlic and onion. Remove from the heat.
2. Combine the garlic and onion with the meat, salt, and pepper. Do not overhandle the meat. Form into 3 patties.
3. Preheat the grill to high. Coat the burgers with olive oil and place on

the grill. Cover and reduce the heat to medium. Allow about 4 minutes per side, turning once.

OR

Coat a skillet with olive oil and heat to medium. Place the meat in the skillet and fry about 2 minutes on each side. Serve.

OPTIONS
- Good with sauteed mushrooms, tomato slices, or grilled onions.

Adapted from a recipe courtesy the American Ostrich Association.

Herb Marinated Ostrich Steak

VERY LOW CARBOHYDRATES　　　　　　　　　　　**NUMBER OF SERVINGS: 3 OR 4**

⅓ **cup balsamic vinegar**
2 tablespoons olive oil
1 tablespoon garlic, finely chopped
½ **tablespoon rosemary, crushed**
½ **tablespoon thyme**
½ **teaspoon black pepper**
1 pound tender ostrich steaks, about 1½
　　inches thick

1. Combine the vinegar, olive oil, garlic, rosemary, thyme, and pepper in a plastic bag. Add the meat and close the bag. Place in the refrigerator for 1 hour, turning occasionally.
2. Preheat the broiler to high.
3. Remove the meat from the marinade and discard the marinade. Place on a broiler pan; position the pan under the broiler 3 or 4 inches below the heat.
4. Broil 2 to 3 minutes, turning once. Meat will be medium-rare to medium.
5. Remove from the broiler, cut into slices, and serve.

Recipe adapted from one developed by Spice Islands Good Harvest test kitchen, courtesy of the American Ostrich Association.

Grilled Rabbit

TRACE OF CARBOHYDRATES   **NUMBER OF SERVINGS: 4 TO 6**

1 large rabbit, cut into serving pieces
Salt and pepper
½ cup sherry cooking wine
½ cup olive oil
1½ teaspoons seasoned salt

1. Preheat the grill on high.
2. Sprinkle the rabbit pieces with salt and pepper.
3. Combine the wine, oil, and seasoned salt.
4. Place the rabbit pieces on the grill. Baste with the wine and oil mixture. Close the lid and reduce the heat to medium. Turn the pieces and baste frequently. Rabbit is done in about 1 hour.
5. Remove from grill and serve.

I wanted to experiment with rabbit, but I was having trouble finding a source. The many dozens of rabbits dancing around our farm gave me an idea. I invited friends over for a rabbit supper with a P.S. "Bring your gun." They laughed, but have yet to show up for a meal!

Turtle Fricassee With Wine

VERY LOW CARBOHYDRATES   **NUMBER OF SERVINGS: 4 TO 6**

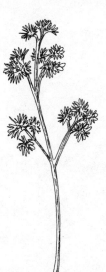

2½ to 3 pounds turtle meat
Salt
Red pepper
2 tablespoons olive oil

½ cup white cooking wine
¼ cup onion, chopped
3 tablespoons butter
Juice of 1 lemon
1 teaspoon minced fresh parsley
1 teaspoon tarragon
¼ teaspoon dried thyme leaves

1. Rinse the turtle pieces and pat dry with paper towels. Sprinkle with the salt and red pepper.
2. Heat the olive oil in a large skillet over medium heat. Put the meat in the skillet and brown on all sides, about 10 minutes. Reduce the heat to low.

3. Drain off the oil. Add the remaining ingredients. Cover and simmer for about 45 minutes, or until tender.
4. Serve.

OPTIONS
- Delicious served with a green salad.

Adapted from a recipe courtesy Seattle's Finest Exotic Meats, Inc.

Exotic Blues Burger

VERY LOW CARBOHYDRATES   **NUMBER OF SERVINGS: 2**

1 pound ground exotic meat: kangaroo,
buffalo, ostrich, venison, alligator, elk
2 teaspoons House of Blues Seasoning Mix
(see recipe below)

1. Preheat the grill to high heat.
2. Combine the ground meat and the seasoning; form into burger patties.
3. Place the meat on the grill. Close the lid and reduce the heat to medium. Turn the meat once, halfway through. Cook to desired doneness.

For Exotic House of Blues Seasoning Mix, combine:

¼ cup kosher salt
1 tablespoon + 1 teaspoon dried onion
flakes
1 tablespoon granulated garlic
1 tablespoon basil
1 tablespoon thyme
1 tablespoon oregano
1 tablespoon black pepper

OPTIONS
- Serve topped with lettuce, tomato slices, and your favorite cheese.

Adapted from a recipe courtesy Seattle's Finest Exotic Meats, Inc.

Sauteed Dijon Exotic Burgers

VERY LOW CARBOHYDRATES   **NUMBER OF SERVINGS: 2 OR 3**

> 1 pound ground exotic meat: buffalo,
>   kangaroo, ostrich, or venison
> 1 egg
> 1 tablespoon dried celery flakes
> 2 tablespoons finely diced onion OR 1
>   tablespoon dried onion flakes
> 2 tablespoons Dijon mustard
> 1 tablespoon balsamic vinegar
> ¼ teaspoon coarsely ground black pepper
>
> 1 tablespoon olive oil

1. Mix all of the ingredients but the olive oil. Form into patties about 1-inch thick.
2. Heat the olive oil in a skillet. Cook the burgers over medium heat for about 4 minutes per side, until just cooked through.

OPTIONS
- Serve with lettuce, tomato, dill chips, diced onion, Westbrae Unsweetened Un- Ketchup, or mustard.

Adapted from a recipe by Russell McCurdy, President, Seattle's Finest Exotic Meats, Inc

Untraditional Irish Stew

LOW CARBOHYDRATES   **NUMBER OF SERVINGS: 5 OR 6**

> 2 pounds of a choice meat: venison,
>   buffalo, cobra, alligator, ostrich
> 1 tablespoon juniper berries, crushed
> 1 tablespoon black peppercorns
> 2 garlic cloves, coarsely chopped
> 1 cup dry red wine
>
> 2 to 3 tablespoons olive oil
>
> 2 cups celery, cut into 1-inch diagonals
> 6 to 8 small boiling onions, peeled
> ¾ to 1 cup beef stock
> ½ cup additional dry red wine

Exotic Meats   287

Salt and pepper as desired
½ cup freshly hand-picked shamrocks (for garnish)

1. Remove all connective tissue and/or fat from your selected meat. Cut into 1-inch cubes.
2. Using a non-aluminum bowl, combine the meat, juniper berries, peppercorns, and garlic. Add the 1 cup of red wine. Cover and marinate in the refrigerator for 2 to 3 hours, or overnight.
3. Preheat the oven to 350°.
4. Drain off the marinade and discard. Heat the olive oil in a heavy skillet over high heat and brown the venison.
5. Add the celery and onions and stir-fry a bit.
6. Add the additional ½ cup red wine and ¾ cup beef stock. Cover and bake in the oven for 45 minutes, or until the meat is tender. Add the remaining beef stock during baking, if necessary.
7. Remove from the oven and season with salt and pepper to taste.
8. Serve garnished with shamrocks and have a happy St. Patrick's Day!

This recipe courtesy Ryan Larsen, Manager, Seattle's Finest Exotic Meats, Inc. Thanks, Ryan!

Appendices:

No-Carb/Low Carb APPETIZER IDEAS

Canadian Bacon

Spread with prepared mustard-horseradish mixture; roll up, fasten with a toothpick, and broil until lightly browned.

Bologna

Spread 5 slices of no-carb bologna with Philadelphia Cream Cheese sprinkled with chives; place layer upon layer. Cut into pie slices.

Chipped Beef

Spread with Philadelphia Cream Cheese sprinkled with chives. Roll tightly and chill. Cut the roll into thirds and serve. Tuck a tiny sprig of parsley in each end.

Stuffed Celery

½ cup Philadelphia Cream Cheese, 1 teaspoon onion juice, and paprika. Spread on small pieces of celery sliced diagonally.

Bacon-Oyster Wraps OR Bacon-Olive Wraps

Cut 8 slices of bacon into thirds. Wrap each third around a canned, smoked oyster that has been tossed in balsamic vinegar OR wrap each third around a stuffed olive. Bake at 375° for 20 minutes. Serve hot.

Bacon-Shrimp Wraps

Cut the bacon in halves or thirds as needed to wrap around small shrimp. Broil.

Pork Rinds

Serve as is or with a cheese dip.

ADAPTABLE RECIPES

The following recipes can be used as appetizers (make the meatballs smaller):

Broiled Italian Beef Burgers, page 21
Speedy Swedish Meatballs, page 26
Savory Swedish Meatballs, page 27
Oriental Meatballs, page 28
Parmesan Meatballs, page 29
Tangy Meatballs, page 30
Easy Chicken Fingers, page 170
Crunchy Chicken Breast Strips, page 171
Stuffed Eggs, page 257
Deviled Eggs, page 257
Marinated Shrimp, page 249
Savory Bison Oven Roasted Meatballs, page 277

Egg Salad Supreme, page 258, can be stuffed in an edible flower, like glads or squash blooms, for a lovely appetizer. (Be certain blossoms have not been sprayed with a pesticide.)

THE BASICS TO Building an Encore Salad Meal

GREENS

There are many to choose from; the **green loose-leaf types** have the most nutrients.

Rinse leaves well and place in a salad spinner OR lay on towels on the counter until nearly dry and then place in a plastic bag in the refrigerator. (I've done bushels and bushels this way, but now much prefer my salad spinner!) I love to get lettuce fresh from my garden, and I raise several kinds for this purpose. There are also many varieties of greens available year round in stores.

PROTEIN

You can use **any cooked protein.** Cut away any bone, fat, or gristle and dice into bite-sized cubes.

VEGETABLES

Favor vegetables with a low glycemic index; these have the least carbohydrates: **celery, cauliflower, broccoli, kohlrabi, mushrooms, asparagus, red and green peppers, onions, zucchini, or a little tomato.**

HERBS

Fresh parsley, cilantro, garlic, chives, or other herbs add flavor, as do dried herbs or blends like Italian Blend Seasoning, etc.

DRESSING

You can purchase very low-carb dressings with no added sugar OR make your own from the **recipes following** or included throughout this book.

TOPPINGS

Cheese can be wonderful. Try grated Parmesan, shredded cheddar, mozzarella, Swiss, etc. Also consider topping with **a few nuts** that have been lightly toasted—pecans, almonds, cashews, macadamia, walnuts, etc. You might try a crumbling a few **pork rinds** for a crunchy, no-carb croutons replacement.

GARNISHES

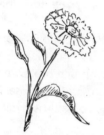

Besides the usual **sprig of parsley, radish rose, green onion or green or red pepper slice,** try using a single **strawberry** or **a few pomegranate seeds**—or how about freshly-picked **violets** (mine grow wild in my flower beds and have white, lavender, or purple blossoms) OR raise **edible flowers,** like nasturtiums, bachelor's buttons, snapdragons, squash (which are also great sauteed in butter), hibiscus, pansies, or daylilies OR use just the flower petals from roses, calendula, carnation—even dandelions (which grow wild everywhere, and the dandelion leaves can be added to the salad greens).

Note: DO NOT experiment with a pretty blossom unless you are certain it's safe to eat; some are poisonous. And DO NOT take plant material from a lawn or garden that has been treated with chemicals unless the label specifically states that it is safe to ingest.

Another garnish idea: Take a small ball of **Philadelphia Cream Cheese**, roll it in chopped chives, nuts, or pork rinds, and place on top of a salad.

If you are using the salad for a meal, remember that all the elements are there to enhance the protein, not overwhelm it, and that the protein should be the main ingredient.

The following recipes contain no, or very low, carbohydrates. The carb count is per one 2-tablespoon serving.

Easy Oil & Vinegar Dressing
(also called French Dressing)

> ¾ cup olive oil OR oil of choice
> ¼ cup wine vinegar OR cider vinegar OR
>   herb vinegar
> 1 teaspoon salt
> ¼ teaspoon pepper

1. Place in a tightly covered jar and shake. Serve over the salad.
2. Store unused dressing in the refrigerator.

OPTIONS

• Sprinkle salad with Italian spice seasoning blend OR herb blend of choice.
• Sprinkle a little minced garlic OR gingerroot over the oil and vinegar on the salad.
• Place a clove of garlic in the dressing bottle.

Mustard Vinaigrette Dressing

> ½ cup olive, sesame, or safflower oil
> ⅓ cup cider vinegar (buy one with no carbs)
>   OR wine vinegar
> 1 tablespoon Dijon mustard OR Grey
>   Poupon
> 1 tablespoon water OR lemon juice (1.3
>   grams carb)
> 1 teaspoon black pepper

Place all of the ingredients in a small container with a tightly sealing lid and shake well.

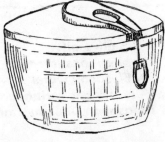

Encore Salads   **293**

1 garlic clove, minced
½ teaspoon basil
½ teaspoon dried chives
¼ teaspoon salt

Place all of the ingredients in a small container with a tightly sealing lid and shake well OR use a Cusinart hand blender with blade.

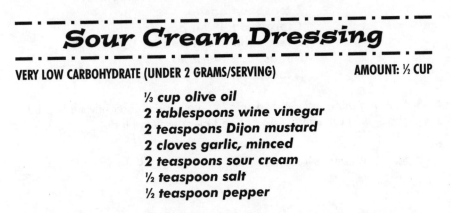

Sour Cream Dressing

VERY LOW CARBOHYDRATE (UNDER 2 GRAMS/SERVING)   **AMOUNT: ½ CUP**

⅓ cup olive oil
2 tablespoons wine vinegar
2 teaspoons Dijon mustard
2 cloves garlic, minced
2 teaspoons sour cream
½ teaspoon salt
½ teaspoon pepper

Place all of the ingredients in a small container with a tightly sealing lid and shake well OR use Cuisinart Hand Blender with blade.

Paprika Dressing

TRACE CARBOHYDRATES   **AMOUNT: 1¼ CUPS**

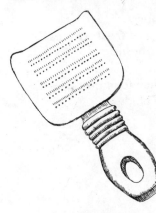

⅔ cup olive oil
¼ cup red wine vinegar
1½ tablespoons water
1 tablespoon Dijon mustard
2 teaspoons paprika
½ teaspoon salt
½ teaspoon minced gingerroot
¼ teaspoon pepper

Place all of the ingredients in a small container with a tightly sealing lid and shake well OR use Cuisinart hand blender with blade.

OPTIONS

• Add 1 teaspoon of poppy seeds.
• Substitute ¼ teaspoon dry ginger + 2 tablespoons Westbrae Unsweetened Un-Ketchup— really good; adds 2 grams total carb.

Italian Dressing

TRACE CARBOHYDRATES   **AMOUNT: 1¼ CUPS**

¾ cups olive oil
2 tablespoons balsamic vinegar
2 tablespoons red wine vinegar
1 teaspoon basil
1 teaspoon onion powder
1 teaspoon black pepper
¼ teaspoon oregano
¼ teaspoon salt

Place all of the ingredients in a small container with a tightly sealing lid and shake well OR use Cuisinart hand blender with blade.

OPTIONS

• Substitute raspberry vinegar for the red wine vinegar.

Russian Dressing

TRACE OF CARBOHYDRATES   **AMOUNT: ABOUT 1 CUP**

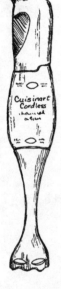

1 cup Hellman's Original mayonnaise
1 tablespoon Westbrae Unsweetened Un-
    Ketchup
¼ teaspoon chili powder
1 to 2 teaspoons chopped fresh chives
2 teaspoons canned pimento

Place all of the ingredients in a small food processor OR use a Cuisinart hand blender with blade.

Poppy Seed Dressing

LOW CARBOHYDRATES   **AMOUNT: ABOUT 1½ CUPS**

> 1 cup olive oil
> ¼ cup lemon juice
> ¼ cup vinegar
> 1 teaspoon salt
> ½ teaspoon dry mustard
> ½ teaspoon paprika
> ½ teaspoon poppy seeds

Place all of the ingredients in a small container with a tightly sealing lid and shake well OR use a Cuisinart hand blender with blade.

OPTIONS

- Instead of the poppy seeds, substitute caraway seeds, celery seeds, dill seeds, or sesame seeds.

Cooked Creamy Caesar-Style Dressing

TRACE OF CARBOHYDRATES   **AMOUNT: ABOUT ⅔ CUP**

> ½ cup cooking oil
> 1 clove garlic, crushed
> 2 egg yolks
> 2 tablespoons wine vinegar
> 2 tablespoons lemon juice
> ¼ teaspoon dry mustard
> ⅛ teaspoon Worcestershire sauce

1. Combine the oil and garlic in a jar with tight-fitting lid. Refrigerate several hours or overnight. Remove the garlic. Set oil aside.
2. In a small saucepan over very low heat, cook the remaining ingredients, stirring constantly, until the mixture thickens and bubbles at the edges. Remove from heat. Let stand to cool, 5 to 20 minutes.
3. Pour the saucepan mixture into the reserved oil. Cover and shake until well-blended OR pour into a blender container, add the reserved oil, cover, and blend at high speed until smooth.
4. Cover and chill if not using immediately.

Recipe courtesy of the American Egg Board.

EQUIPMENT Sources

The Baker's Catalogue
P.O. Box 876
Norwich VT 05055-0876
800 827-6836
www.kingarthurflour.com
Fine tools, ingredients, equipment, and books for the home baker. My nutmeg mill, cinnamon mill, and Quick Whip came from here. They stock my very favorite stainless steel measuring spoons, long and thin enough to fit into spice jars. Now I've got my eyes on their hanging cookbook holder!

Camerons Professional Smoking Products
CM International Inc.
P.O. Box 60220
Colorado Springs CO 80960-0220
Phone: 888 563-0227
Fax: 719 390-0946
www.cameronsmoker.com
Ask for their great Stovetop Smoker and wood chips at gourmet cooking shops; you can call them for the store nearest you. They're also coming out with other products; check their Web Site. The Stovetop Smoker is available by mail from Chef's Catalogue, below. A must-have!

Chef's Catalog: Professional Restaurant Equipment for the Home Chef
P.O. Box 620048
Dallas TX 75262
800 338-3232
www.chefscatalog.com
All kinds of great equipment, including knives, pots and pans, Cuisinart and KitchenAid small appliances, Cameron's Stovetop Smoker Cooker, and even Weber grills. Scoops for meatballs come in four sizes.

A Cook's Wares: Superior Gourmet Gifts and Supplies
211 37th St.
Beaver Falls, PA 15010-2103
800 915-9788
www.cookswares.com
Fabulous pans, bakeware, cutlery, appliances, and utensils plus wonderful herbs, spices, oils, and vinegars.

Kitchen & Home
P.O. Box 2527
La Crosse WI 54602-2527
800 414-5544
www.kitchenandhome.com
A wide variety of wares from fish poachers to vertical rotisseries and even tablecloths and dishes. I'm especially fond of their dripless, smokeless candles, which allow me to entertain without worrying about smoke allergies.

PCD: Professional Cutlery Direct, for the Chef's Essential Tools
170 Boston Post Road, Suite 135
Madison, Connecticut 06443
Phone 800 859-6994
Fax: 800 296-8039
www.cutlery.com
More than just knives, this nice little catalogue also offers high-quality cookware, pepper mills, and utensils. I'm coveting their new kitchen scale!

Weber Grills
P.O. Box 1999
Palatine IL 60078-1999
Phone: 800 99-WEBER (800 999-3237)
Fax: 847 705-7971
www.weberbbq.com
Wonderful barbecue grills and equipment—we love our Weber!

FOOD Sources

Allen Brothers—The Great Steakhouse Steaks . . . delivered right to your door
3737 South Halsted Street
Chicago, IL 60609-1689
Phone: 800 890-9146 Fax 800890-9146
www.allenbrothers.com
Besides beef, veal, lamb, pork, turkey, and chicken, they also stock Scottish smoked salmon, lobster tails, and jumbo shrimp.

Dean & Deluca—Purveyors of Fine Food and Kitchenware
560 Broadway
New York NY 10012
Orders: 800 221-7714
www.dean-deluca.com
Premium proteins like fresh Norwegian salmon, smoked eel, live lobsters, smoked goose breast, Cornish hens, cheeses, the finest quality spices, vinegars, and oils.

Denver Buffalo Company: The Flavor of the New West
P.O. Box 480603
Denver, CO 80248-0603
Phone: 800 289-2833
Fax 800 278-7100
www.denverbuffalo.com
Their catalogue features quite an extensive array of buffalo.

Heartland Selections
P.O. Box 7527
Kansas City, MO 64116-0227
Phone: 800 827-2867
Fax 800 299-3573
www.farmland.com—"See Shopping Aisle"
Boneless pork chops, marinated pork tenderloins, filet mignon, Kansas City Strip steaks, etc.

Jackson Hole Buffalo Meat
P.O. Box 2100
Jackson Hole, WY 83001

www.jhbuffalomeat.com
They specialize in the finest hickory-smoked 100% buffalo meat products.

Omaha Steaks
10909 John Galt Blvd.
Omaha, NE 68137
Phone: 800 960-8400
www.omahasteaks.com
Marketer of steaks and other frozen gourmet foods.

Penzeys, Ltd. Spices and Seasonings
P.O. Box 933
Meskego, WI 53150
Phone 414 679-7207
Fax 414 679-7878
www.penzeys.com
Their catalogue features a mouth-watering assortment of herbs, spices,
and blends—and seasonings are an important part of keeping protein
dishes interesting.

**Seattle's Finest Exotic Meats, Inc. "All Natural Farm Raised
Exotic Meats From Around the World—No Hormones, No
Additives, All Natural"**
17532 Aurora Ave, North
Seattle WA 98133
206 546-4922 800 680-4375
www.ExoticMeats.com
They offer alligator, antelope, buffalo, caribou, cervina, cobra, duck,
rabbit, rattlesnake, snapping turtle, squab, venison, wild boar, and wild
turkey for sale and their web site has many recipes.

Wooden Nickel Buffalo Farm, Inc.
5970 Koman Rd.
Edinboro, PA 16412-3902
814 734-BUFF (ALO) or 2833
www.woodennickelbuffalo.com
USDA inspected bison meat.

Wyoming Buffalo Company
1280 Sheridan Ave.
Cody, WY 82414
800 453-0636
www.wyobuffalo.com
Catalog available with over 400 foods and gift items; they feature gourmet Western foods.

CARB COUNTS
for Ingredients

Almonds, slivered, ¼ cup = 9
Anchovy paste, 1 teaspoon = 0.3
Apple juice, 1 cup = 29.5
    1 5½ ounce can = 19
Apple, 2¾-inch diameter = 20
Artichokes, 14-ounce can = 27
Asparagus, fresh, 4 spears = ¼ pound = 2.2
Avocado, 1 medium = 12
Bacon, Canadian, fried, 1 slice = 0.1
Bacon, Hormel, fried, 2 strips = 0
Bamboo shoots, 1 cup = 7.9
Basil, 1 teaspoon = 0.9
BBQ Spice Blend, purchased, 1 teaspoon = 1.0
Bean sprouts, mung, 1 ounce = 1.9
    1 cup canned = 1.5
Beef roast = 0
Beef steak = 0
Beefer-Upper, info not available
Beens, green, 1 cup = 6.8
    Fresh, French style, 3½ ounces = 3.4
Beer, Miller Lite, 12-ounce can = 3.2
Bison, roast, 3½ ounces = 0
Bouillon, granulated, 1 teaspoon = 1
    1 cube = 1.4
Bourbon, gin, 1 ounce = trace
Brandy, 40 percent alcohol = trace
Broccoli, 1 cup, raw = 7
    cooked = 8.5
Broth, beef or chicken, canned = 0
Butter, 1 stick or 8 tablespoons = 0.5
Buttermilk, 1 cup = 12.5
Cabbage, shredded, 1 cup, raw = 4.9;
    1 cup, cooked = 6.2
Capers, 1 teaspoon = 0
Caraway seeds, 1 teaspoon = 1
Carrot, 1 large, raw = 7

1 large, cooked = 11
Cashews, 18 nuts = 8.3
   ½ cup, whole = 16
Cauliflower, 1 cup, raw = 4.4;
   1 cup, cooked = 5.1
Celery salt, 1½ teaspoon, estimated = 0.8
Celery seed, 1 teaspoon = 0.8
Celery, raw, 1 cup = 3.9
Cheese, American, 1 ounce = .5
   cheddar, 1 ounce = .6
   Monterey jack, 1 ounce = 0.2
   mozzarella, 1 ounce = ¼ cup = 1
   Parmesan, grated, 1 ounce = 1 tablespoon = .2
   Philadelphia Cream Cheese, original, 2 ounces = 2 tablespoons = 1
   Romano, 1 ounce = 1; 4 ounces = 1 cup, grated
   provolone, 1 ounce = 1
   Romano, 1 ounce = 1 gram
   Swiss, ¼ cup = 1 ounce = .5
Chicken = 0
Chili powder, 1 teaspoon = 1.4
Chives, 1 tablespoon, fresh = .6
Cilantro, 1 teaspoon, dried = .3
Cinnamon, 1 teaspoon = 1.8
Coconut, 4 tablespoons = 2
   fresh, shredded, ½ cup = 6.8
Cognac, 40% alcohol = trace
Coriander, ground, 1 teaspoon = 0.5
Cottage cheese, 2 percent milkfat, ½ cup = 3
Cream, heavy whipping, 1 tablespoon= 0.6
   1 cup= 9.6
   ½ cup= 4.8
   ⅓ cup= 3.2
   ¼ cup= 2.4
Cumin, 1 teaspoon = 0.9
Curry powder, 1 teaspoon = 1.2
Dandelion greens, 1 cup = 6.7
Diet pop = 0
Dill pickle chips, 1 ounce = 1
Dill seed, 1 teaspoon = 1
Dill weed, dried, 1 teaspoon = .6
Eggs, medium hard-boiled, 1 = 0.5
Egg yolk, 1 = 0.1
Fennel seed, 1 teaspoon = 1.1
Fish, plain = 0
Garlic powder, 1 teaspoon = 2.0
Garlic, raw, 1 clove = 0.9

Ginger, 1 teaspoon = 1.3
Gingerroot, fresh, 1 ounce = 3
    1 teaspoon = 0.5
Goose = 0
Grapes, 1 cup = 27.7
    10 grapes = 8.7
Ground beef = 0
Ham = 0 (check the label!)
Herbs and spices, 1 teaspoon, dried = 1 or 2
Horseradish, 1 tablespoon = <1
Hot dogs = 0 (but check the label!)
Kitchen Bouquet, 1 teaspoon = 3
Kohlrabi, raw, ½ cup = 4.3
    cooked = 5.5
Kumquat, 1 medium = 3
Lamb = 0
Lemon juice, 1 tablespoon = 1.3
    1 whole medium lemon = 3 tablespoons juice = 5.4
    zest, 1 teaspoon = .3
Lemon pepper, 1 teaspoon = 1.0
Lettuce, romaine, 1 cup = 1.9
    Boston or Bibb, 1 cup = 1.4
    iceberg, 1 cup = 1.6
Lime juice, 1 tablespoon = 1.4
    1 whole medium lime = 2 tablespoons juice
    zest, 1 teaspoon = 0.3
Macadamia, 6 nuts = 2
Mace, 1 teaspoon = .9
Marjoram, 1 teaspoon = 0
Mayonnaise, Hellman's Original = 0
Mushrooms, fresh, 4 ounces = 1 cup = 3.1
      10 mushrooms = 4.4
    canned, Giorgio's, ½ cup = 3
      4 ounce can = 1 cup = 6
Mustard, Dijon, 1 teaspoon = 1
    dry, 1 teaspoon = .3
    regular yellow, prepared, 1 teaspoon = .3
Nutmeg, 1 teaspoon = 1.1
Nuts, 4 ounces = ¾ cup, chopped = 1 cup ground = 20
Olive oil = 0
Olives, green with pimento, Lindsay 5 = <1
    black, sliced, 3.5-ounce can, drained = 14
    2 tablespoons, sliced = 1
Onions, green, chopped with tops, ½ cup = 3.7
      1 tablespoon = 0.9; ⅓ cup = 2.2
    powder, 1 teaspoon = 1.7

dried flakes, 1 tablespoon = 4.2
raw, chopped, ½ cup = 6.9
    1 medium = ¾ cup, chopped, = 8.7
    1 tablespoon = .9
Orange zest, 1 teaspoon = .5
Oranges, mandarin, Dole, ½ cup = 19
Oregano, 1 teaspoon = 1
Paprika, 1 teaspoon = 1.2
Parsley, 1 tablespoon = .3
Peach, fresh, 2¾ inch diameter = ½ cup, diced = 4.8
Pecans, ¼ cup pecan or pieces = 5
Pepper, black, 1 teaspoon = 1.4
    red, whole, 1 medium = 8.0
    green bell, diced, raw, 1 cup = 1 whole pepper = 7.2
    Jalapeno chili, 4.5-ounce can = 3
    red sweet, diced, raw, 1 pepper = 1 cup = 10.2
    red cayenne, 1 teaspoon = 1.0
    white, dried, 1 teaspoon = 1.7
Pepperoni, Oscar Meyer, 15 slices = 0
Pimento, 4 ounce jar = 6.6
Pineapple, juice, 6-ounce can = 22
    1 ounce = 2 tablespoons = 3.7
    1 cup canned in water = 25.1
Pomegranate, 3½ inch diameter = 25.3
Pork = 0
Pork rinds = 0
Pork sausage, 1 ounce = 0.3
Poultry seasoning, 1 teaspoon = 1
Radish, 1 large = 0.29
Raisins, dark, 2 tablespoons = 15
Rosemary, 1 teaspoon = 0.8
Saffron, 1 teaspoon = 1
Sage, 1 teaspoon = 0.4
Salad dressing, Hain French creamy, 1 tablespoon = 0
Salsa, Tostitos, 2 tablespoons = 3
Sauerkraut, 1 14-ounce can = 33
Scallions, 1 tablespoon = 0.5
Scallops, steamed, 3½ ounces = 1.8; raw = 3.3
Sesame oil = 0
Sesame seeds, 1 tablespoon = 1.4
Shallots, 1 average clove, finely diced = 1 tablespoon = 2.5
Sour cream, 1 tablespoon = 1
    1 cup = 8 ounces = 16
Soy sauce, 1 tablespoon Kikkoman = 0
Spinach, raw, 1 cup = 2.4
    cooked = 6.5

Squash, summer, 1 cup, cooked = 6.5
Summer sausage = 0 (check the label!)
Swiss chard, 1 cup = 4.8
Tabasco Sauce = 0
Tarragon, 1 teaspoon = 0.8
Thyme, 1 teaspoon = 1
Tomato, 1 fresh, 2.6-inch diameter = ½ cup = 5.8
    sauce, Hunt's, ¼ cup = 3
        8-ounce can = 1 cup = 10.5
    cooked, 1 cup = 13.3
    Hunt's, canned in juice, ¼ cup = 4
        14-ounce can = 14
    crushed in juice, Mrs. Grimes, 14.5-ounce can = 15
Turkey = 0
Turkey = 0
Vermouth, 3½ ounces = 1
Vinegar, Balsamic, wine, cider, tarragon, 1 tablespoon = .9
Walnuts, ¼ cup = 5
Water chestnuts, ¾ cup = 11
Water = 0
Westbrae Unsweetened Un-Ketchup = 1 tablespoon = 1
Whiskey, 40% alcohol = 80 proof, 1 fl. ounce = trace
Wine, burgundy, 1 cup = 24
    sherry cooking, Holland House, 2 tablespoons = 2
    red cooking, Reese, 2 tablespoons = 3
    Chablis cooking, 2 tablespoons = 3
    white cooking, Holland House, 2 tablespoons = 0
    Burgundy cooking, Reese, 2 tablespoons = 3
Worcestershire sauce, Heinz, 1 tablespoon = 0
Zucchini, ½ cup = 1.9
    boiled = 3.5

SOURCES

Atkins, Dr., *Dr. Atkins' New Carbohydrate Gram Counter*. New York: M. Evans and Company, 1996.

Netzer, Corinne T., *The Complete Book of Food Counts, 3rd Edition*. New York: Dell Publishing, 1994.

Pennington, Jean and Church, Helen, *Food Values of Portions Commonly Used, 14th Edition*. Philadelphia: J. B. Lippincott Company, 1985.

United States Department of Agriculture, *Nutritive Value of American Foods in Common Units Agricultural Handbook No. 456*. Washington, D.C.: United States Department of Agriculture, 1975.

Also consulted nutritional information available on food packaging.

Acknowledgments

To the many people who've dined at our house, willing guinea pigs for my relentless experimenting, most particularly the Fehrs: Randy, Jane and especially Berneice; their constant love and encouragement are most appreciated—

To those who went before me: my mother, my grandmother, my Swedish great grandmother, and my "adopted" Aunt Nell, fine cooks all; their influence is present in this cookbook—

To George de Kay, with affection, for his friendship and uncommon good sense—

To Dr. Atkins, with gratitude, for teaching the truth about nutrition, and—

To you, the reader, for making this book a success. Here's to your good health as you dine on wonderful food!

About the Author

Barbara Doyen was born and raised in Iowa, America's heartland where beef, pork, and poultry are produced. She is married to a farmer who has raised much livestock, though he now concentrates on grains like corn and soybeans.

A serious cook, the author preferred near-vegetarian/low-fat cuisine years before the current fad, making all her own foods from scratch. Upon the advice of a doctor, she prepared even stricter vegetarian low-fat foods to counteract her husband's high cholesterol and blood pressure. But his condition continually worsened as did her own low blood sugar problem—until she changed to a protein-based diet with higher fat content as described in books like *Dr. Atkins' New Diet Revolution*. The improvement was dramatic.

Currently running her own literary agency from a country acreage, Barbara Doyen comes from a background in education (as a K-12 art instructor for 15 years) as well as television (writing and appearing in her own weekly series on commercial TV for one year). She has authored many instructional materials for writers, including an audiotape series endorsed by James Michener. An active 4-H member while growing up, her cooking demonstration won a trip to the state fair, earning a blue ribbon. Now she is frequently invited to do speaking engagements and demonstrations and her well-received WRITE TO $ELL seminars have helped thousands of beginning and experienced authors further their writing careers.

Visit the author at barbaradoyen.com

Index